Swimming for Life

THE THERAPY OF SWIMMING

RONALD RUSSELL

PELHAM BOOKS
STEPHEN GREENE PRESS

PELHAM BOOKS/STEPHEN GREENE PRESS
Published by the Penguin Group
27 Wrights Lane, London W8 5TZ, England
Viking Penguin Inc., 40 West 23rd Street, New York, New York 10010, USA
The Stephen Greene Press Inc., 15 Muzzey Street, Lexington, Massachusetts 02173, USA
Penguin Books Australia Ltd, Ringwood, Victoria, Australia
Penguin Books Canada Ltd, 2801 John Street, Markham, Ontario, Canada L3R 1B4
Penguin Books (NZ) Ltd, 182–190 Wairau Road, Auckland 10, New Zealand

Penguin Books Ltd, Registered Offices: Harmondsworth, Middlesex, England

First published 1989

Typeset in 11/13pt Concorde by Goodfellow & Egan Ltd, Cambridge
Printed and bound in Great Britain by Richard Clay Ltd, Bungay, Suffolk

British Library Cataloguing in Publication Data

Russell, Ronald
    Swimming for life: the therapy of swimming
    1. Physical fitness. Swimming
    I. Title
    613.7′1

ISBN 0-7207-1860-0

Contents

The illustrations to Chapter 5 are by Ulla Frisch.

Preface

To be asked to write the Preface to this important book is both a privilege and a joy. Having been in close contact with the author during the long period of research and data collecting, I can speak of his dedicated persistence in journeying up and down the United Kingdom to inspect facilities and to interview people connected with swimming at all levels. The result is the most important assembly of facts and experiences yet presented concerning this natural yet neglected alternative therapy.

Until reading this book I had the idea that I knew something about swimming and its use as a therapy. Now I am aware of how ignorant and ill-informed I have been.

As the years rolled by and my attention turned more and more to the search for simpler and more effective alternatives to the costly and limited orthodox therapies, I had neglected as a way of healing – or should I say 'wholling' – what was perhaps my own favourite sport. I had neglected what is perhaps the most natural and all-encompassing alternative approach, truly 'whole person directed' rather than symptom or syndrome adapted as so much of present-day 'alternative' therapy has become to its detriment.

Reading Chapters 1 and 3 made me shudder to think how many people I could have helped to better use of themselves and so to a fuller life over my fifty years of practice, had I simply turned them to Nature's own gentle and easily available healing to relearn movement and breathing in the supportive element of water.

It is with these personal regrets in mind that I suggest with all my heart that every medical practitioner, every specialist, every therapist, reads, ponders and uses the data presented in this vade-mecum of *Swimming for Life*.

Put swimming first on your list of alternatives. It is yoga in water!

Professor A.T. Andreasen FRS(E) FRSC(E) FICS

The First Length

An Introduction

Swimming for Life derives from observation and experience. To live with someone who is in constant pain, cannot walk more than half a mile, cannot sit in a chair for more than ten minutes, who wears a surgical collar and whose arm and leg muscles are usually wrapped in bandages is an experience for both observer and observed which they may well feel they could do without. But then, five years later, to see that same person swimming eighty to a hundred lengths a day before beginning several hours intensive physical work massaging other people's bodies, spending holidays walking in the Yorkshire Dales, shaking off infections and other problems at a moment or two's notice, and at the same time raising some £30,000 for various charities by swimming – that experience validates the earlier one and makes the pattern whole.

'I'm sorry, but there's nothing more we can do for you. You'll have to learn to live with it, I'm afraid. We can let you have as many painkillers as you want, of course, but that's about all.' These will be familiar words to many people. You may find them depressing and disheartening. They hold out no hope, no prospect that things might ever improve. You have been sentenced to a lifetime of suffering with no hint of reprieve or remission. You have defeated all the resources of medical science, and this is your reward.

But you do not have to take the words in this way. 'There's nothing more we can do for you' does not mean that there is nothing that you can do for yourself. You can, for example, seek for help in other directions. There are many approaches other than the one adopted by orthodox Western medicine; perhaps one of them will be more suited to deal with your particular difficulty. You can look for health – and health is far more than simply absence of disease – in places other than a hospital. One of these other places is a swimming pool.

Of course it is not as simple as that. Swimming does not provide a 'miracle cure' any more than Yoga, acupuncture, homeopathy or chemotherapy would do. Swimming is first of all a sport, an enjoyable recreation. Most of us swim for fun, not for our health. If we 'feel better' afterwards that is a bonus, but it is not the reason why we go for a swim.

Is there then any difference between swimming for fun and swimming for health? In one important respect the answer is 'No'. If you do not find it fun it will not do you much good. Apart from that, however, it is largely a matter of will. If you swim only for fun, you do not go unless you feel like it. If you swim for health, you swim whether you feel like going or not. You swim regularly and for much of the time energetically, developing a consistent breathing pattern, adding up the lengths, trying always to swim as well as you can, freeing your mind from daily worries. It will also be fun.

Observations and experience prove this to be the case, and samples of these are given in *Swimming for Life*. They were gathered through a series of interviews and through questionnaires distributed via swimming clubs and organizations, the swimming press, a number of osteopaths (who are especially interested in swimming and other forms of exercise as therapy) and many helpful individuals.

It matters to know also what opportunities are available, in particular for disabled or handicapped people or those who are rehabilitating after illness or injury. Many elderly people who have not visited a public pool since they splashed about in an effort to keep warm in the stark municipal baths of their youth are deterred from indoor swimming by their grisly memories. They need to know that conditions have improved and that most pools nowadays have quiet periods in which old folk can find out how swimming suits them now.

You do not need to be ill to swim for your health. Swimming is best regarded as a type of preventive medicine, or as an efficient means of keeping your body in good physical condition – or helping to return it to that condition after injury or illness. As the Health Education Council says: 'Although you inhabit an electronic, push-button, high-technology world, you still have a Stone Age body.' This body developed to survive in a harsh physical world and it continues to need physical activity to keep it trim and in good working order. Regular energetic exercise lessens the risk of heart disease and helps to control weight and release tensions. Everyone knows this, but few pay it more than lip-service.

While governments boast of the amount of money spent on the Health Service, the demands on the Service seem continually to increase. Waiting lists extend over months, staff are overworked, outpatients' departments and doctors' waiting-rooms are crowded, and the whole massive organization is under constant stress. Part of the solution lies not in providing yet more money and costly equipment but in extending and developing the concept of health education, shifting the responsibility for wellness to the individual, working far more energetically towards the prevention of illness rather than merely seeking to deal with it when it occurs. The Health Education Department should be central to the Service, not lingering on the periphery as it usually is. More swimming pools and other sporting facilities, with people shown how to use them intelligently and consistently – and encouraged to continue using them throughout their life-span – would do much to alter attitudes towards health and illness and to free hospitals to deal with the real emergencies, the more drastic problems, for which they are best suited.

Within a few days of completing the second draft of *Swimming for Life* I heard that Professor Andreasen had died at the age of seventy-nine. The idea for the book was his; he kept a careful eye on its progress, made many helpful and stimulating suggestions and contributed the typically modest and generous Preface.

Tony Andreasen enjoyed a long and distinguished career as an orthopaedic surgeon both in England and overseas. During this career he developed a deep interest in alternatives to technologically oriented routines. He came to see the pursuit and maintenance of health as a partnership between practitioner and patient using one or more of several available methods, and as a search, for both of them, for the essential inner balance without which spiritual and physical harmony cannot exist. Characteristic of his unifying way of approach is the visualization technique described in Chapter 2.

Tony's personal experience of the value of swimming derived from his practice of swimming long distances daily in the tideway in his youth and was enhanced more recently by observing the effects of regular swimming on the progress of one particular patient. This led him to encourage the writing of *Swimming for Life*, which is dedicated to him with respect, gratitude and love.

—1—

Swimming as Therapy

Recognition of the therapeutic value of regular swimming is nothing new. In 1764 Dr E. Baynard wrote a poem entitled *Health* which included the following lines:

> Of exercises, swimming's best,
> Strengthens the muscles and the chest,
> And all their fleshy parts confirms.
> Extends and stretches legs and arms,
> And, with a nimble retro-spring,
> Contracts, and brings them back again.
> As 'tis the best, so 'tis the sum
> Of exercises all in one,
> And of all motions most compleat,
> Because 'tis vi'lent without heat.

Much earlier, in hearty classical times, both Homer and Virgil referred to the healthy properties of swimming. In *The Aeneid* Virgil makes Numanus describe how:

> Strong from the cradle, of a sturdy brood,
> We bear our new-born infants to the flood;
> There bathed amid the stream our boys we hold,
> With winter hardened and inured to cold.

Today in Soviet Russia a similar policy is pursued, except that there one-month-old infants are taken to bathe in warm pools in children's clinics, with, it is said, the result that they grow up essentially healthier and much less prone to infection.

In ancient Rome and the surrounding towns and villages there are estimated to have been about 850 public baths. Some of them were equipped with gymnasia, spaces for ball games, a variety of pools maintained at differing temperatures and various other amenities, and they seem remarkably like antecedents of our present sports and leisure centres, except that the Roman establishments were more generously staffed. Julius Caesar was a strong swimmer, though apparently less strong than Cassius; Seneca preferred chilly rivers to warm water; and Horatius's swimming ability saved his life. The Romans gave the highest priority to swimming as an exercise and the daily plunge was virtually a duty for all citizens.

Among the Anglo-Saxons and the Vikings swimming seems to have been an activity for heroes whose prowess inspired admiration, but in later centuries its importance diminished. It became a gentlemanly accomplishment but not a particularly important one. References in literature are few and far between until the latter part of the sixteenth century when Richard Mulcaster devoted a whole chapter to swimming in *Positions* (1581), where he dealt specifically with its benefits for health, including making the joints 'nimble' and improving the digestion. He warned against the dangers of 'exhalations' from the water and came out strongly in favour of swimming in the sea. Six years later Everard Digby wrote *De Arte Natandi*, which was abridged and translated by Christopher Middleton in 1595 as *A Short Introduction for to learne to Swimme*. It was described as the first scientific treatise on the subject and its influence lasted for two hundred years.

When he wrote his book, Digby was a clergyman, philosopher and a Fellow of St John's College, Cambridge, although he was expelled from the college later following controversy over his religious views. He enjoyed outdoor life and became concerned at the numbers of young men who died from drowning in the rivers and lakes near Cambridge. One motive for the book was to give instruction in swimming in order to save lives and another was to establish the status of swimming as an art. He maintained that swimming promoted health, in which respect it is compared to medicine, 'especially as the fittest thing to purge the skin from all external pollutions or uncleanness whatsoever, as sweat and such like, as also it helpeth to temperate the extreme heat of the body in the burning time of the year'. From the instructions and illustrations it can be seen that stroke-making at the time was rudimentary – he describes a dog-paddle, a sort of breaststroke, something like an Old English backstroke and a sidestroke which he says is the fastest though the most laborious. Of equal importance are various acrobatic poses, such as showing four parts of the body above the water at once, swimming with one hand and one foot upon the back, and cutting toenails in the water!

At least two well-known treatises on swimming in the following decades were plagiarized from Digby but it was not until the nineteenth century that any significant advances in instruction were made. Joseph Strutt's *The Sports and Pastimes of England* (published 1801) included only one page on swimming with the vague comment that 'in London we are told two centuries back there were men who could teach the art of swimming well'. Then in 1816 a swimming teacher from Nottingham, J. Frost, wrote *Scientific Swimming*, 'a series of practical illustrations on a progressive plan by which the art of swimming may readily be attained, with every advantage of power in the water'. Things were now beginning to move; a National Society on the Art of Swimming was formed, which published two prize essays on the subject in 1841. Nevertheless, as late as 1857, B. C. Richardson, author of *Instructions in the Art of Swimming*, did not believe that a quarter of a mile had ever been swum in a quarter of an hour but that a man might swim a hundred yards at a speed equivalent to a mile an hour at best. However, this was the age of improvement; several books on swimming and allied subjects appeared in the middle years of the nineteenth century (including three on baths and wash-houses between 1852 and 1854) and the sport began to be studied in a more scientific and methodical manner. Among the more thoughtful publications were *A Manual of Swimming, including Bathing, Plunging, Diving, Floating, Scientific Swimming, Training, Drowning and Rescuing*, by Charles Steedman, 'Champion of England and Victoria', and *The Swimming Instructor* by William Wilson. Later in the century the founding of the Amateur Swimming Association and the consequences of the passing of the Baths and Washhouses Act in 1846 led to a firmer structure for the sport and enabled far more people to participate.

In 1893 the volume entitled *Swimming* in the Badminton Library of Sports and Pastimes was published. Over 400 pages in length, this was the most comprehensive study yet to appear. The authors, Archibald Sinclair and William Henry, believed that swimming should be part of the national education. 'It is generally admitted,' they wrote, 'that the pastime has great advantages over all others, and that it is a most pleasant and suitable form of bodily exercise, and most important for the preservation and promotion of health. It has a beneficial influence on the blood and its circulation. Bodily exercise, when taken judiciously, is indisputably good, and many of the disturbances in the digestive organs to which mankind is now so prone would be avoided if swimming and bathing were more generally practised.' The authors also commented on the beneficial effects of swimming on the respiratory system, adding that 'the strengthening of the digestive organs tends to increase the muscular and mental capacities of men, thereby proving the truth of the old adage *Mens sana in corpore sano*'. But they were critical of the legislature for failing to realize the value of swimming apart from its usefulness in the saving of life at sea. They concluded their reflections by forecasting that 'the time may come when the reproach that one can neither swim nor read will be considered as indicative of a notorious dunce as it was in the days of Aristotle.'

The literature on swimming has increased vastly during the present century, especially since about 1960, although compared with other major sports there is little available in print at any one time. Mostly it consists of instructional books, of which by far the most significant is James E. Counsilman's *The Science of Swimming*, first published in the USA in 1968 and reprinted many times. Counsilman deals mainly with competitive swimming at the highest level – he was a highly successful Olympic coach – but much of the book is of great value and interest to swimmers of any ability.

For swimming as therapy perhaps the most comprehensive study is *Adapted Aquatics*, compiled by the American National Red Cross and published in the USA in 1977. Subtitled 'Swimming for persons with physical or mental impairments' this was founded on the experience of the American Red Cross in developing swimming programmes for handicapped veterans from World War II. These programmes were developed and extended in the following years and *Adapted*

Aquatics was published as the textbook for Red Cross instructors' courses, designed 'to be a resource for all persons working with the handicapped in swimming programmes'. The book is fully illustrated and as well as chapters on 'Impairments and Disabilities', 'Facilities and Equipment', 'Competitive Opportunities' and 'Programming' it also includes material on behaviour modification and academic reinforcement through aquatics. The authors make two very important points that the enthusiastic organizer or instructor might easily overlook: one emphasizes the fun element in the various swimming activities, and the other warns against the tendency to categorize or label individuals according to their handicaps, thus focusing attention on disability rather than ability.

The value of swimming, both physiologically and psychologically, for disabled people and those rehabilitating after accident, illness or injury is widely acknowledged by the medical profession. In *Swimming Medicine*, vol. 4 (published in 1978 and incorporating the proceedings of the Fourth International Congress on Swimming Medicine held in Stockholm) the following list of disorders was given for which swimming is 'recommended therapy':

> arthritis, blindness, cerebral palsy, diabetes mellitus, epilepsy, mental retardation, muscular dystrophy, multiple sclerosis and multiple handicaps.

Swimming was recommended to restore and maintain fitness in instances of chronic obstructive pulmonary disease, ischemic heart disease (including myocardial infarction), obesity, poliomyelitis and sports injuries generally. Finally, swimming is considered beneficial in the following conditions:

> amputations, ankylosing spondilitis, intervertebral disc disease, juvenile discogenic disease

(Scheuermann's), scoliosis, kyphoscoliosis, spondylolysis, spondylolisthesis, spina bifida, traumatic paraplegia and tetraplegia, and asthma.

Nevertheless it is surprising how few of those who have recorded their experiences for this book were recommended to swim by their doctors. Consulting room dialogue, usually constricted by time, is often, it seems, confined to the point of pain and the prescription pad, while many hospital doctors are apparently oblivious to what their patients do when discharged from hospital or released from the out-patient clinic. If the suggestion comes from the patient, the doctor may well agree with it, but it seldom seems to apply the other way round. Yet there are very few people who will not benefit from swimming and very few physical or mental conditions for which swimming is contra-indicated.

Osteopaths, on the other hand, have swimming in the forefront of aids to recovery. Of the eighty osteopaths whose opinions were sought for this book, every one recommends swimming to patients for whom it is thought it would be appropriate. Osteopathy is concerned with maintaining and restoring the balance of the neuro-musculo-skeletal system, using manipulative therapy and no drugs. Treating far fewer patients than a general practitioner, an osteopath can devote much more time to diagnosis and management and has more opportunity to discuss the patient's life-style and occupational strains.

The condition most commonly treated by osteopaths is 'backache', which is the second most frequent cause, after bronchitis, of lost working hours. Other complaints treated include sports injuries, pain and restricted movements in joints and head, postural and mobility problems (including arthritis), digestive troubles, gynaecological difficulties, migraine, asthma, occupational stress and tension states. Osteopaths treat mainly with the hands and recognize that what the patient does between treatments is often as vital as the treatment itself. This is where exercise, and particularly swimming, becomes an essential part of the healing process for a remarkably wide variety of conditions. 'I always recommend swimming unless the condition makes it impossible or dangerous,' says one practitioner. 'Swimming is the only exercise I recommend to my patients because there is very little chance of doing any harm and a great potential for improving health,' says another.

However, the simple recommendation 'You should try swimming', may by itself prove of little help. This is especially true for people with musculo-skeletal problems where discrimination between different swimming strokes and attention to stroke technique are likely to be of importance. For certain spinal conditions the over-use of breaststroke may prove harmful, and those with neck trouble who use this stroke but do not put their faces in the water may accentuate their problems. Back crawl is generally suitable but may be inadvisable for people with certain shoulder conditions. A knowledge of correct technique is necessary and lessons in swimming would be of value as part of the training of osteopaths – and sensible and useful for medical students as well.

Swimming may be recommended to help rectify a particular condition, especially where weight-bearing should be avoided. Some practitioners, however, adopt a rather different approach, summed up in the words of one: 'I am more concerned to promote the idea that swimming involving exercise of the whole body with deep breathing promotes health of all tissue. I do not expect much symptomatic improvement in the short term.' The vital importance of breathing technique is echoed by others:

I advocate swimming to aid breathing patterns in asthmatics, fat people, unfit people. This is done in conjunction with teaching patients to breathe using their diaphragms more effectively.

and,

I place emphasis on correct control of breathing while swimming, especially in the exhalation phase, e.g. during forward thrust in breaststroke with face in the water.

and,

Swimming is excellent for breath control.

Unfortunately the medical profession at large pays little attention to breathing patterns or mechanics, seeming to regard breathing as something that just happens naturally and can be left to look after itself. Professor Andreasen takes a different view:

To breathe is to live. Quality of Life is proportionate to the effectiveness of the breathing pattern, its range, rate and rhythm. A quick way of proving this is to get a (very good) friend to hold your head under water until you fight free to get that Breath of Life. There is nothing like Experience! . . . Than breathing there is no more important function. All else depends upon it. Delay in taking up breathing rhythm can mean brain damage for the neonate. Inefficient breathing during life means poor brain function and therefore poor mind/body response to environmental impact, both external and internal – hence disorder, distress and disease.

The personality and attitude of the patient is as relevant here as it is – or should be – in all areas of treatment. One practitioner said: 'I only recommend swimming for people who enjoy it. No benefit is derived if it is treated as a penance.' It was generally felt, however, that swimming was more popular than most other forms of exercise, although deterrents were reported:

> A number of patients avoid swimming where it might otherwise be suitable because (a) water too cold – even in indoor pools (but this may be an excuse!) and (b) a lack of opportunity when the pool is free from crowds of children in school parties.

and,

> Unfortunately English 'heated' swimming pools are not that warm; also the pf balance is irregularly attended to, resulting in stinging eyes, etc. These put a lot of people off. Also crowds and distance to travel.

Sometimes the patient himself presents the deterrent: 'Regular swimming requires commitment and many patients will not even do simple exercises at home.' But on the whole it seems to be the 'abysmal local facilities' in some areas that prevent more people from enjoying what most practitioners agree is a highly beneficial form of exercise. Chilly water, crowded pools and the failure to set aside reasonably convenient times for adults only or serious swimming are the chief criticisms. It is also true, however, that many doctors and osteopaths are unaware of the local provision for swimming and of the various incentives and award schemes that are available.

The general conclusions from the survey of osteopaths may be summarized as follows: All osteopaths recommend swimming to their patients where they think it is appropriate. Swimming is most frequently suggested for the following conditions:

a range of lower back problems, muscular or spinal
in origin;
asthma, bronchitis and allied problems;
many arthritic conditions;
degenerative or inflammatory joint conditions.

Swimming is also recommended for:

general health and fitness;
recovery after accident, injury or long confinement
to bed;
improved fitness during and after pregnancy;
improved cardio-vascular and muscle tone;
degenerative conditions where non-weight bearing
exercise will help;
challenging lazy patients to help themselves get
better and not expect the practitioner to do all the
work for them.

Relevant to this last point, and also to the futility of
self-deception where health is concerned, is the comment of one practitioner who is himself keenly aware of
the value of swimming as a remedial exercise:

A lot of people tell me they 'keep fit' by swimming
and yet I know that they only move gently up and
down the pool with no great effort and therefore
no increase in their 'fitness'. It is obviously better
than no exercise, but my own opinion is that one
has to increase lung capacity, strengthen the heart
and reduce pulse rate with a reduced recovery
period to be achieving fitness. None of these can
be achieved without some degree of effort. I feel a
lot of people deceive themselves by thinking that
you can get 'fit' by swimming because it requires
less effort.

A further comment on technique comes from an
osteopath who was himself a competitive swimmer:

I have observed when swimming myself that a
significant number of people swim with very
incorrect techniques, e.g. screw-kick in breaststroke. I wonder therefore if some patients are not
gaining maximally from their exercise because of
asymmetrical use of joints and muscles and the
detrimental effect this has on musculo-skeletal
mechanics. I wonder whether patients to whom I
recommend swimming who come back to me and
say that their condition was aggravated have not a
technical problem with their strokes.

For the best possible therapeutic effect a swimming
programme should be devised for the individual
patient, who should be told if any strokes are to be
avoided and directed to take advice from a swimming
teacher or coach on the efficacy of his stroke technique.
Distances should be increased gradually and the individual must accept that a degree of effort is required if
he is hoping for positive results. And, lastly, a word to
anyone thinking of swimming for the sake of his or her
health: if you don't enjoy it, don't do it – you'll merely
be wasting your time.

It is interesting to note that swimming is highly
regarded as a beneficial activity in the practice of yoga.
For teachers and followers of yoga, correct breathing is
by far the most important factor in the pursuit and
maintenance of health. In *Yoga and Health*, a widely
popular and influential book on what might be called
'Western Oriental Yoga', Selvarajan Yesudian and Eli-
sabeth Haich devote a chapter to 'Swimming: for perfect breath regulation'. They point out that swimming is
a natural exercise, not an artificial one, and that 'it is the
only sport in the world which, because of the perfectly
rhythmic movements required, forces us to breathe
deeply in the pranayama manner.' ('Prana' can be
loosely rendered as 'cosmic energy', and 'pranayama' as

'the conscious practice of controlling prana through concentration and regulated breathing.') As swimming forces you to control your breathing it can be treated as a form of yoga exercise. Certain techniques are suggested: in breaststroke inhaling, then taking two long strokes with the face in the water and exhaling through the nose on the second stroke; and in the crawl taking four strokes with the face immersed and exhaling powerfully towards the end of the cycle. Clearly this will be even more beneficial if you are swimming in the open air.

2

Swimming for All

To improve your general health and physical condition, and to maintain this improvement, you should regard swimming as part – though a very important part – of an overall fitness programme. You are primarily responsible for your own health, as any given society is primarily responsible for the health of that society, no matter how small or large it may be. Unless that responsibility is acknowledged and acted upon, progress will be slow, if it happens at all, and suffering may be needlessly prolonged.

Advances in hygiene and medical science have, in Western civilizations, destroyed many of the old destroyers such as cholera, smallpox and tuberculosis. We live in a cleaner and wealthier age than ever before. Nevertheless many diseases continue to flourish; cancer, diabetes, atherosclerosis and heart disease among them. These and other characteristic degenerative diseases of the twentieth century are caused principally by what we – as individuals and as members of society – do to ourselves. The damage caused by smoking is now generally recognized to the extent that it is at last becoming a socially unacceptable practice, harmful to others as well as to the smoker himself. In recent years eating habits have been more closely scrutinized. 'Over half of the more common forms of cancer are related to diet which makes the combined effect of food and drink the most important determinant of the risk of cancer,' said Dr Jan de Winter, founder and first Director of the Whole Body Scanner Department at the Royal Sussex County Hospital. The authors of *Clinical Ecology*, Dr G. T. Lewith and Dr J. N. Kenyon, even advocate the avoidance of processed food of all sorts and recommend that the use of aerosol sprays, garden pesticides, weedkillers and artificial fertilizers should be banned.

The last few years have seen an increasing interest in 'alternative' therapies. Many towns and cities now have Natural Health groups providing information about a range of therapies including acupuncture, homeopathy, chiropractic, herbalism and many others. To some extent this interest is the consequence of disillusionment with orthodox medicine in the shape of the National Health Service with its crowded waiting-rooms, lengthy hospital waiting lists, exclusive use of chemical drugs, and its poor public image. But no single therapy, alternative or orthodox, has a monopoly of wisdom; the most that any therapy can do is to put the individual into a position or state of mind where he or she is best able to assist or accept the body's own healing power and process. For some the general practitioner or hospital consultant may provide the most effective help; for others it may be the osteopath or yoga teacher. But by itself no therapy can be fully effective. Patient and practitioner need to work together, each with a willingness to listen and learn, to enable the mind/body's powers of recovery to operate with maximum efficiency.

There has been an avalanche of major advances in medical technology in the past few decades. Hospital floors groan under the weight of massive items of diagnostic machinery. Developments in fibre optics enable surgeons to see where previously they could only deduce or guess. Transplant surgery is becoming almost commonplace and is dependent on the avail-ability of donor organs rather than on the numbers of trained surgeons. Preventive medicine, on the other hand, has made far less progress than was envisaged in the early days of the Health Service, and Health Educa-tion remains a poor relation of the Service, underman-ned and under-resourced. Sometimes the transplant surgeon is called on to replace what the patient himself has caused to become diseased. At great expense, technology and human skills are employed to deal with a condition that might have been prevented. This is all too often the way of things.

As far as most people are concerned, however, the most effective preventive medicine is within their own grasp. 'Exercise is the best therapy in the world; it can prevent more diseases and it can solve more problems than any medicine yet developed,' says Dr de Winter. 'Regular exercise is one of the best ways of eliminating poisonous waste products that have accumulated in the body, thereby restoring the proper balance in the blood of its many essential constituents. Additionally, physi-cal exercises tend to release pent-up emotions and thereby relieve mental stress.' Exercise has three main physical functions: to improve the circulatory and res-piratory systems, to develop mobility in muscles and joints, and to increase muscular strength and tone. Of all exercise activities, swimming performs these func-tions in the most effective and satisfying way.

The advantages of swimming are many. It exercises the whole body, not just bits of it. Supported by the water, joints and muscles move freely, unhampered by gravity and protected from the jarring and knocking that can happen in land-based exercise. In the horizon-tal attitude blood-pressure is lowered and in water the risk of heat exhaustion is greatly diminished. The rhythmic movement and the gentle massaging of the

Choosing your exercise

(from the Health Education Council's booklet *Looking after Yourself*)
Remember, whatever you choose to do, always *go easy* to start with and build up *gradually*.

S-FACTOR SCORE

	Stamina	Suppleness	Strength
Badminton	**	***	**
Canoeing	***	**	***
Climbing Stairs	***	*	**
Cricket	*	**	*
Cycling (hard)	****	**	***
Dancing (ballroom)	*	***	*
Dancing (disco)	***	****	*
Digging (garden)	***	**	****
Football	***	***	***
Golf	*	**	*
Gymnastics	**	****	***
Hill Walking	***	*	**
Housework (moderate)	*	**	*
Jogging	****	**	**
Judo	**	****	**
Mowing lawn by hand	**	*	***
Rowing	****	**	****
Sailing	*	**	**
Squash	***	**	***
Swimming (hard)	****	****	****
Tennis	**	***	**
Walking (briskly)	**	*	*
Weightlifting	*	*	****
Yoga	*	****	*

* No real effect   *** Very good effect
** Beneficial effect   **** Excellent effect

And do not expect miracles overnight. It will take at least three twenty-minute sessions of vigorous exercise each week for about six weeks before you really notice the benefits.

water puts the mind at peace. Marianne Brems, an American Masters national record holder, expresses this same notion eloquently: 'When you swim you escape into a cool silent world where you have only your own motion, your own breathing, and your own thoughts enveloping you in a way that is nothing like life on land.'

The Health Education Council rates swimming as the top exercise for stamina, suppleness and strength. It is one of the few sports that can be enjoyed regardless of age and, to a great extent, regardless of physical disability as there are very few conditions where swimming is contra-indicated. It is also comparatively cheap with little equipment needed and most pools providing reduced rate season tickets for regular swimmers. Indoor heated pools are not affected by the weather and many of them are open from early morning until late evening so it should be possible to find a time when there are no crowds and you can swim as you wish.

Most modern pools are 25 metres in length; a few are 33 metres and a very small number are longer still. If you are not used to swimming it is best to begin by trying a few widths, moving to lengths as soon as you feel sufficiently confident. Concentrate on achieving a smooth and relaxed style, keeping the body as streamlined as possible and as nearly parallel to the surface of the water as you can manage. Get used to swimming with your face in the water, turning or lifting your head only to inhale, and be prepared to wear goggles to protect your eyes and provide clearer vision. Breathe deeply in time with the stroke action and do not worry about speed until you have thoroughly mastered the strokes.

For positive physical – and mental – benefit you need to swim reasonably energetically, without stopping, for a good ten minutes. Visit the pool twice a week (more often if you can) and remain in the water for at least twenty minutes. Try to master breaststroke, backstroke and front crawl and use at least two of them on each swim as each makes demands on different joints and muscles. Build up speed and distance gradually, setting time and distance targets every now and then to measure progress. Do not be discouraged by muscular youths who swim three or four lengths while you are completing one; remember that if you had enjoyed their opportunities when you were that age you would doubtless have done just as well – or even better.

A general exercise programme is valuable whether you are a swimmer or not. There are several suitable books on the market to advise you, usually illustrated by lithe, supple, perfectly proportioned figures far removed from those that most of us see in the bedroom mirror. It does not matter much which programme you choose provided that you listen carefully to what your body is telling you and stop when it says it has had enough. Unless you have special instructions from a physiotherapist or osteopath, concentrate on exercises that stretch the muscles, improving flexibility and mobility; the rolling, bending, swinging, twisting, flexing movements. At the beginning and end of each session, breathe in deeply, using the muscles of the diaphragm and raising your arms on either side. Then exhale hard, dropping the arms and shoulders and bending forwards to squeeze all the breath out of you. Repeat three or four times. When you have finished the session, rest for a few minutes before doing anything else.

As well as a general programme there is a set of simple exercises, especially designed for swimmers, which are aimed at strengthening the muscles mainly employed in swimming. These are quite demanding and intended for reasonably fit and active people. Do not try them all at once but build up gradually, adding a new exercise every two or three days until you have managed all seven. A session of between ten and fifteen minutes should be enough for anyone.

For maximum benefit from these exercises you should follow a basic breathing pattern. This is quite simple and once established it can be carried over into all forms of physical activity:

> Exhale when making an effort.
> Inhale on the recovery phase.

This will ensure rhythm and eliminate forced and jerky movements.

Examples of the exercises are as follows:

a) Lie face down, legs together, toes tucked under, hands under shoulders with fingers facing forwards. Straighten your arms so that you are balancing on hands and toes, keeping back and legs still and rigid. Lower down gently and repeat, building up with practice to ten moves.

b) From the straight arms position in (a) jump forward to squat, balancing on toes and palms with your knees outside your elbows. Then kick back to the previous position. This exercise is familiar to watchers of television's *Superstars*.

c) Lie on your back, legs together, knees slightly bent, hands linked at back of neck. Sit up, leaning forward until your head touches your knees. Return slowly to the first position.

d) Sit with knees bent and feet tucked under your backside. Put your hands on the ground behind you and lean back, raising your knees to stretch your ankles.

e) Stand with arms raised to shoulder level in
    front of you. Keeping them at this level, pull
    them hard back to the sides. Repeat several
    times.

f) Stand as in (e) with palms down. Swing arms
    up and back in as large a circle as possible.
    Repeat several times.

g) Put some chalk on the index finger of one
    hand. Stand sideways to a wall, the chalked
    hand nearest. Bend knees slightly and leap
    into the air, raising both arms and marking
    the wall with chalk at the top of the leap.
    Leave the mark and try to beat it the next
    time.

It is helpful to know what actually happens when you
are swimming, both inside your body and in the water
around you. The physiological effects, which provide
solid evidence of the value of swimming as a health-
promoting activity are dealt with clearly and concisely
in the Amateur Swimming Association's very useful
book *The Teaching of Swimming*. The long-term
effects, which occur as 'a result of systematic but
carefully monitored overloading of the body during
regular performance' can be summarized as follows:

improvement in the proportion of muscle to fat;
strengthening of connective tissues (cartilages,
    ligaments, tendons) and intermuscle and
    organ supporting tissue;
increase in the tidal volume of the lungs;
improved blood supply to the lungs and to the
    heart muscle itself;
increase in size and strength of the heart,
    leading to a lower normal heart rate;

increase in the number of capillaries;
increase in the haemoglobin and number of the
    blood cells;
improved efficiency in muscle and all tissues
    and organs in extracting oxygen from the
    blood as well as discharging the products of
    their living processes into the venous drainage
    side of the circulatory system.

The word 'overloading' indicates that if you want these benefits you have to work for them. You may not be training for a race but you are training your body to respond more effectively to the strains and stresses placed upon it daily throughout your life.

Certainly, of equal importance is the ability to relax whilst swimming. Physically this means using the minimum amount of energy while moving with the greatest possible rhythm and precision. 'Better relaxation', say the authors of *The Teaching of Swimming*, 'and consequent improved efficiency result from swimming progressively longer distances without stopping. Although a stroke may be quite poor technically, it can still be relaxed. Improved relaxation results in a reduction of the energy expended and so a greater distance can be swum. This in turn can lead to further improvements in technique and in relaxation.'

Mental relaxation is no less important. Several of our swimmers talk of 'throwing their worries into the pool' and coming out with minds free of anxieties and uncluttered by trivia. To begin with, your mind should be fully occupied with what you are doing: controlling your breathing pattern, improving your rhythm, polishing your technique and checking your balance. Try not to be distracted by what other people are doing and follow your own course. Then, when all feels right, let your mind go. Sometimes it helps to count strokes or breaths, or to repeat a single word or a mantra. 'It's like meditation,' said one of our respondents; 'you are in your own world and no one can reach you.' This is what has been described as 'the Yoga of Swimming'.

If this peaceful state of mind is not easy to come by, there is a simple visualization technique which may help:

1. Before entering the pool relax totally for a few minutes, breathing deeply.
2. See yourself swimming freely, moving and breathing rhythmically and easily and feeling happy and at peace.
3. Get up quickly and enter the water, holding this visualized sense of total rhythm and ease.
4. Continue to swim in this frame of mind. Do not strive or compete or allow yourself to be distracted.
5. Having finished your swim, retain the awareness of quiet ease and total rhythm until you come to swim again.

Understanding what goes on in the water around your body helps you to improve your stroke technique and hence to enjoy your swimming more. 'A swimmer must use not only his body but also his mind; this is what makes swimming such a challenging and enjoyable activity,' wrote Dr Counsilman in *The Science of Swimming*. To improve your performance you need to decrease resistance, caused by the water through which you are moving, and to increase propulsion, created by the effects of your arms and legs. Understanding how to achieve these aims is the basis of success. For immediate and practical purpose we can simplify this by looking to the example of streamlining vehicles or aircraft in order to diminish the resistance of the air through which they move. Man's body in relation to water is about as streamlined as a Model T Ford, but enormous improvements can be made by altering the angle of the swimming body in relation to the water surface. The smaller the angle, the more effective the streamlining; the straighter your body and the nearer your feet are to the surface (without breaking it) the faster you will move for the same expenditure of energy. Dropping the legs or failing to point the toes when the legs are extended will slow you down, as will lateral body movements or excessive rolling from side to side. You can learn much about this by watching other swimmers, not from the pool side but while swimming yourself wearing goggles and observing them with your head submerged.

Propulsion drives you forward through the water and is created by your hands and arms, and sometimes by your legs and feet, as they pull you forward, pushing the water behind you. An understanding of Newton's three laws of motion may help you to appreciate the principles involved, but his third law – that to every action there is an equal and opposite reaction – is the one most relevant to progress in swimming. Fortunately, you do not need to go into the technicalities of hydrodynamics or fluid mechanics to become a good swimmer, although they will be very helpful if you simply want to become a good swimming coach. As swimming is an activity where it is comparatively easy to judge one's own progress you may learn a great deal by experimenting for yourself to discover the best type of pull, the most effective hand position and the most efficient kick and how to incorporate your breathing into the stroke cycle. Every now and then, however, it is valuable to look over the stroke mechanics as described in a good swimming manual or, better still, to have a session with an experienced coach or swimming teacher. This will ensure that you do not fall into bad habits and that you are getting the best possible returns from your expenditure of energy.

Most swimmers begin with the breaststroke. This stroke provides forward vision and most people find it comparatively easy to make the arm and leg movements coincide in a regular and symmetrical fashion. Do not try to emulate competitive breaststroke swimmers who lift most of the upper body clear of the water during the stroke cycle but concentrate on trying to achieve a smooth and flowing forward movement. You can swim breaststroke with your head above water all of the time and you will see many people doing so. This is, however, inefficient and places strain on the muscles at the back of the neck. The most effective head position is with the water-line about mid-forehead, raising the head just sufficiently to inhale through the mouth and lowering it to exhale under water. Much of the propulsion comes from the leg kick and this stroke is especially useful if you wish to strengthen your leg muscles.

Front crawl is the fastest stroke, with continuous propulsion and the least resistance. Here the face is submerged nearly all the time, with inhalation on either side at whatever stroke interval the swimmer finds most efficient. The legs serve to stabilize the body rather than to contribute to forward movement; hence the stroke makes its demands mainly on arm and shoulder muscles. The noisy splashing progress through the water that some swimmers make is not to be imitated; a smooth, flowing movement is far more effective and can be sustained for a much longer time.

Most swimmers enjoy swimming on the back, either as the preferred stroke or as a change from crawl or breaststroke. The back crawl is the competitive method and the most popular; here you use an alternative overarm action and a flutter kick – very much the reverse of front crawl. Alternatives are the elementary backstroke, in which the arms do not break the surface but perform a sculling action while the leg kick resembles a breaststroke kick the other way up, and the

English backstroke with a similar leg action and the arms swinging back simultaneously. The face is out of the water throughout and it is sensible to develop a suitable breathing pattern so as not to fall into the habit of breathing too rapidly and shallowly.

The butterfly developed from the breaststroke; the arms and the legs act simultaneously, giving intermittent surges of power but no continuous forward progress. To swim this stroke effectively demands much physical strength but the splashing and heaving that often accompanies its performance make it generally unsuitable for a crowded swimming pool. However, it does suit some swimmers, particularly those whose movements are instinctively symmetrical and who therefore are naturally adept at breaststroke. Most coaches consider that you need to be able to swim front crawl well before attempting butterfly as the breathing patterns are similar.

Other swimming strokes include the front paddle and sculling on the back, both feet-first and head-first, essential in lifesaving practice. There are two varieties of sidestroke, one with a sort of sideways breaststroke action and the other with an overarm recovery out of the water. And you may find someone swimming the Trudgeon – the only stroke called after the name of its inventor – an overarm stroke with the head out of water, popular towards the end of the nineteenth century.

If possible, you should aim for competence in breaststroke, front and back crawl. Anything else is a bonus. And aim to perform these strokes as well as you possibly can; this will provide both satisfaction and a sense of achievement, so helpful in building confidence. 'With intelligent hard work,' says Dr Counsilman, 'each can achieve the best that is within him, and this is the standard he will be measured by, both by other persons and himself.'

A Sussex osteopath has devised a swimming stroke of special benefit to people with weak knee joints, enabling them to exercise without the problems caused by weight-bearing. He describes it as follows:

> The idea is to lie on the back in the water and use the feet and hands as paddles propelling the water away from you, the right hand and foot being synchronized and similarly the left. The knee is slowly flexed and strongly extended. On the outward stroke the sole of the foot is at right angles to the leg and on the inward stroke the toes are pointed to reduce friction as the knee is brought up ready for the next thrust. Similarly with the hand – the water is pushed away with the palm of the hand at right angles to the forearm and drawn back with the hand feathered to reduce friction. The elbow has to extend and flex to achieve this objective. There is a tendency to keep the bottom low in the water of course, but this is a mistake because it slows progress. It is surprising how fast this stroke can become when practised and one can be as vigorous or as gentle as one wishes. I call it the back pedal stroke.

Try also to master the turns appropriate to your strokes. It is not practical to describe these; the best way to learn is through a lesson with a coach, or you can teach yourself by closely observing the practice of good swimmers. Efficient turns at the end of each length make the swim more enjoyable; the stroke rhythm is maintained and the exercise is uninterrupted.

Diving is a specialized skill and not related to fitness except that you need to be fit to do it properly, but it is useful to be able to make a good smooth entry into the water by means of a modified version of a racing start. Again, watch the experienced swimmers and adopt the method that suits you best.

Swimming competitively, if only from time to time, helps greatly to keep a sharp edge on your performance and provides a valuable incentive. This does not necessarily mean taking part in organized races in front of critical or partisan spectators – in any event, unless you are young and very active there are few opportunities for this. Competing against the clock can be very effective; almost all pools have a clock that is clearly visible from the water and this is often all you need to spur you on to greater efficiency and effort. Informal races with other swimmers can also induce you to draw on your reserves and hence derive more benefit from your exercise. For serious competitive swimming, however, in for instance the Masters' competitions for good class swimmers from twenty-five to seventy years of age competing in age groups, a consistent training programme is essential.

For almost everyone, then, swimming is the ideal form of exercise. It affects the whole body, strengthening muscles and increasing flexibility of the joints; it sets up the requirements for full rhythmical breathing; and it increases the effectiveness of blood circulation and the respiratory system. It can be performed only within an individual's limitations at any given time and hence there is little risk of over-exhaustion. Progress can be easily ascertained by the swimmer himself and is measured in graded phases, important for steady and continual improvement. Swimming can be a solitary or companionable pursuit, enjoyed indoors or in the open air. It is comparatively cheap – or free – and needs little equipment: a swimming costume (preferably nylon and workmanlike rather than 'fashionable' – bikinis are best suited to sunbathing), a cap if you need one and a pair of goggles. Various swimming aids are available for learners of all ages; arm-bands and floats are mostly used, but for children who lack confidence or adults whose approach is tentative or who are weakened by illness, injury or disability it may be worth considering the flotation or bubble jacket which enables you to relax completely while practising strokes and does not hinder your freedom of movement. Flippers can be fun while swimming in the sea and useful when training but otherwise should not be used in a public pool.

There are few occasions when you should not swim. In the interest of others as well as of yourself, keep away from the pool if you have a cold or cough or are feverish. Do not swim if you have an open wound, and check first with your doctor if you are suffering from an eye, ear or skin infection, verrucas or athlete's foot. Do not swim within two hours of a heavy meal. Some asthma sufferers may have trouble in pools disinfected by chlorine but they should have no problems in ozone-treated pools – ask the pool manager about this. Cramp is very unlikely to occur in an indoor heated pool.

You are virtually safe from infection in a swimming pool, thanks to the disinfected water; the danger area, if any, is the changing room. Eyes may be protected by goggles, and ears by thorough drying. The exercise itself causes fewer problems than any other sport, although the odd bump and crash may occur in crowded pools through someone's carelessness. Swimmers in training or who frequently and energetically swim long distances may possibly contract tendinitus – pain in the tendons of the shoulder. Using solely front crawl or butterfly is likely to cause this, which makes a strong argument for varying strokes. Small changes in technique may solve the problem, but if it becomes severe a period of rest is advisable and a word with an orthopaedic doctor or an osteopath. Breaststroke specialists do not escape: the joint that may cause them trouble is the knee, and the solutions are similar. The great majority of swimmers, however, will experience neither of these problems and are far more likely to be aware that joints which may disturb them on land move painlessly and smoothly in the water.

Water is kind to pregnant mothers as well. Swimming, as pregnancy progresses, may be the only form of exercise that remains comfortable at all times. It helps to maintain general fitness, provides valuable relaxation and can be continued right up to the final stages. Climbing in and out of the pool may need extra care but otherwise you carry on as normal, using the strokes that you find easiest with the changing distribution of body weight. You may need to make certain stroke adjustments – and tumble turns may become impractical – but otherwise carry on as long as you can.

After the baby arrives, returning to the pool as soon as possible helps you to regain shape and fitness. Moreover you can take your baby with you. Many pools have parent/baby sessions and the classes at the Crystal Palace Sports Centre in South London accept babies at the age of three months. Before long they are moving independently through the water. Anxious mothers can be reassured that this does not mean they are thrown in and left to fend for themselves, although this method does seem to have some success with Californian infants and puppy-dogs. The programme used at the Crystal Palace classes is described in an inexpensive book, *Babes in the Water*, obtainable from the Amateur Swimming Association.[1]

The best way to improve your own swimming style and technique is to have a few lessons from an experienced teacher or coach. You can also learn a great deal

---

1 Professor Andreasen told me that he taught his daughter to swim from the time she was three months old by letting her cling to his back in a little home-made sling which held her safely. Between six and nine months she began freeing herself from his back and imitating his dog paddle and floating. She progressed in this way, until well before her second birthday she was jumping and diving off the board and swimming a natural type of crawl.

from observing other swimmers, especially below
water. With increasing competition in swimming – the
number of events in the Olympics has doubled in the
last twenty years – and the development of under-water
photography there has come a vast improvement in the
understanding of swimming mechanics and the techniques of coaching. Swimming instructional books are
far better than they used to be and all swimmers will
find they can learn much from them. An annotated list
of some readily available books appears in Appendix D.

The Amateur Swimming Association (ASA) has
developed a swimming fitness programme which provides incentives for the individual swimmer and is easy
to follow. The incentives are in the form of awards for
completing a range of distances in miles, from ten to
five hundred. You simply keep a record of the distance
swum on each visit to the pool, entering it on a log card,
and when you have achieved the required total you are
entitled to the appropriately coloured badge. The Association recommends a programme involving long,
gentle swims (for example 100 metres, 200 metres, 400
metres, 800 metres) and short distance swims (25 or 50
metres) taken at a faster speed. The short swims should
be taken in series, 6 × 25 metres, or 4 × 50 metres, with
a rest between each swim to allow breathing to return
to normal. The programme may also include part practices, using legs or arms only with the non-operative
limbs supported by a float, or crawl practices with the
use of one arm only at a time. Some lengths should also
be devoted to stroke improvement with concentration
on a particular aspect of the stroke.

Two schedules are suggested. The first, for beginners
to the Swim Fit programme, as it is called, is as follows:

3 minutes: gentle swimming used as a
             loosener.

5 minutes:	stroke improvement practice.
10 minutes:	3 × 100 metres, resting one minute after each 100 metres, using favourite stroke.
2–3 minutes:	gentle swimming to finish.

Then there is a more advanced schedule:

5 minutes:	gentle swimming using two strokes.
16 minutes:	2 × 400 metres front crawl, swimming fairly easily; rest 1–2 minutes as necessary after each 400 metres.
6 minutes:	4 × 50 metres legs only, using favourite stroke. Attempt to increase speed. Rest as necessary.
5 minutes:	stroke improvement – breaststroke.
6 minutes:	200 metres arms only, using any stroke other than breaststroke. Gentle swimming.
12 minutes:	6 × 50 metres, using favourite stroke, resting as necessary after each 50 metres. Concentrate on speed of swimming.
3 minutes:	gentle swimming to finish.

Periodically, to boost distance towards an ASA Swim Fit award, devote sessions entirely to full stroke swimming.

For a thorough and controlled Swim Fit programme,

begin with sessions of about twenty minutes a time, twice a week, and build up to sessions of approximately one hour as many times a week as you can manage. It is important not to overdo it in the first few sessions. If you do feel acute discomfort or swimming is followed by headaches, dizziness, chest pains or pins and needles in the limbs you should consult a doctor.

You can discover how hard your body is being made to work and how safe the exercise is by checking your heart rate immediately you stop swimming. Count your pulse for fifteen seconds and multiply by four; convenient places are below the jaw bone two inches from the ear or on the wrist with palm turned upwards. According to your age, the rate should lie between the following limits:

age	rate	age	rate
20	140–170	50	119–145
25	136–165	55	116–140
30	133–161	60	112–136
35	130–157	65	108–132
40	126–153	70	105–127
45	123–148		

If you are below the lower figure, the exercise may be too easy; if above the upper figure, it is too hard.

A point worth emphasizing is that you are never too old to take up swimming. In September 1985 a national newspaper reported that a gentleman of ninety-four had just learned to swim by taking a week's swimming course at a hotel near Exeter. The hotel runs one and two week holiday courses during the year using its own small pool heated to 90°F. Many, though by no means all, of the participants are of pensionable age; they are taught in small groups and use the pool two or three times a day, spending the rest of their time in the usual holiday activities. The organizers believe that in the secure and comfortable conditions they provide almost anyone can learn to swim within a week.[2]

Another recent venture is a project under the auspices of the Manpower Services Scheme of Sport for the Over Fifties. This is called 'Swim Therapy' and aims at teaching older people, some of whom have arthritis or other problems, to swim using the Association of Swimming Therapy's Halliwick method. The programme enjoys five hours of pool time a week and over 300 people have passed through it in the last three years, with eighty on the register at the present time and a waiting list. One of the organizers talks of the 'safe and happy people now enjoying their swimming and feeling a great deal fitter than before'. A few similar schemes are in operation up and down the country but there is room for a great many more.

To complement the swimming and general exercise programme, healthy eating is vital. Processing food and selling it is big business and food advertisements are often compelling and effective. We *are* very much what we *eat*; if we are overweight, constipated, with high blood pressure and likely to die of heart disease, then the odds are that we have created these conditions by what we have eaten over the years. We are encouraged by advertisers to eat crisps, pies, biscuits and cereals coated with sugar – they might as well encourage us to take out plenty of life insurance or join one of the health insurance schemes before it is too late. If our diet is overloaded with fats, sugar and salt then we are undoing all the good that swimming provides – and we might just as well not bother. One of the saddest spectacles today is the lunch hour in a secondary school where the school canteen had gone over to

2 These courses are available at the Long Range Hotel, Whimple, near Exeter, Devon.

A Note on Diving

While entry into the water by diving from the pool side is an acknowledged part of swimming, diving from boards is something different. This is recognized by the modern practice of omitting diving boards from most new pools and constructing separate diving pits. Diving is an exhilarating sport with its own specialized techniques. You need to be fit to master these techniques but diving itself does not contribute to fitness, although it improves confidence and, successfully accomplished, leads to an enhanced sense of well-being.

convenience foods – chips, sausage rolls, pasties and the like, washed down with fizzy drinks.

The importance of a well-balanced diet for the top-flight competitive swimmer is heavily stressed by Dr Counsilman; basically, his recommendations are not very different from what is best for most of us, and he warns against the indulgence in greasy or highly seasoned foods, alcohol and smoking. Useful guidelines for the ordinary swimmer can be found in another Health Education Council booklet *Food for Thought*, which deals in a readily understandable way with the issues involved and gives several useful recommendations. It points out the value of a diet high in fibre and low in fats, sugar and salt, lists many of the high fibre foods and gives the calorie and fat content of a number of popular everyday items. Top of the order for calories and fat is the individual pork pie, followed closely by cheesecake, pork chop, cheese and tomato pizza and

scotch egg. The message is beginning to get across –
note the rise of the baked jacket potato in the snack
market – but there is still a very long way to go before
our eating habits make healthy sense. It is ironic that
hospitals, like many schools, are not in the vanguard of
change but still too often provide the unsuitable or
inedible to those who have little or no choice. Finally, if
you have achieved a balanced diet you should not need
any supplements.

3

Does that mean the Disabled too?

Mourna, now aged twenty-nine, is severely disabled as the result of a car accident. Recently she wrote a paper on 'Sport for All' in which she summed up the importance of sport for *all* people, not just the able-bodied. Coming as they do from someone with experience both as an able-bodied and as a disabled person, Mourna's words carry added significance.

One should not look at disabled people for what they cannot do but rather for what they *can* do. Achievements by the disabled continually seem to surprise the able-bodied, simply because they don't think of them as being *able* to succeed in such a fashion.... What is important is one's performance within one's frame of ability. Everyone has a talent for something in some direction. It is a matter of finding it, nurturing and developing it.

Given the opportunity and the spirit, the disabled can overcome many physical handicaps somehow.... On the one hand, it is up to the able-bodied to allow the disabled to incorporate any game or aspect of sport into their lives if they so wish. On the other hand, it is up to the disabled to show that they too have a need and desire to be involved in sport. Situations ought to be created to allow everyone the opportunity to discover their possible capabilities. In the case of disabled people then to develop their abilities. Remember, people may have disabilities in one way but abilities in other ways.

Sport is one area which can help disabled people psychologically as well as physically. The very fact that they enjoy doing things through the physical is a boost, and somehow crosses the barrier line of being called disabled. People generally think of sport purely in the physical sense, but as everything is controlled by the main switch – the mind – sport has many contributions to make to any person's development.

It should be taken for granted that sport is part and parcel of a disabled person's life. Factors incorporated may include: co-ordination, co-operation, determination, effort, skill, stamina, strength, self-confidence, self-reliance, self-control, suppleness and spirit. So sport should be included in a disabled person's programme and should not be overshadowed by visible – or invisible – disabilities.

Society as a whole agrees with Mourna in general terms and within its financial constraints provides facilities, instructors and so forth.

But in practice many problems arise:

Not enough is done to help the physically handicapped after they leave hospital. The National Health Service can only provide very limited after-care, so it's up to the individual. Quality of life is often overlooked when finance has to be considered. If you are poor you are considered to

have a poor quality of life; if you have some wealth
you have to pay for everything yourself. People
who have become physically disabled due, say, to
a stroke or the consequences of neurosurgery can
expect not to do so well out of the system.

This is the comment of a young woman suffering
from partial paralysis following the removal of a brain
tumour. Finding herself forced to seek her own salva-
tion, as it were, she turned to swimming as a therapy. 'It
has maintained what use I have left,' she says. 'It has
helped me to share with others and to make sure that
once a week all my family gets involved. It builds up
confidence and helps one to recover more quickly from
setbacks.' She is now on the committee of her local
swimming club for the handicapped, determined to
ensure that it is run on business-like lines and is aware
of all its members' needs.

A less than perfect Health Service may provide
unexpected benefits. When the experts can no longer
help you, for whatever reason, you have, if you possibly
can, to take the responsibility yourself. Ultimately, it is
worth re-iterating here, you are your own best healer;
others may guide, suggest, administer or prescribe but
the source of the healing power lies within yourself. The
best that a doctor, or any therapist, can do is to partner
you in the healing process.

One of the things that you can do for yourself – one
of the most helpful – is to swim. The British Sports
Association for the Disabled emphasizes the importance of swimming for disabled or handicapped people,
pointing out that it has long been recognized as their
'premier form of sport and recreation. In swimming the
handicapped are unencumbered by the artificial aids
which are necessary to them for everyday mobility. In
the water it is possible for them to realize that there is a
form of inexpensive and readily available recreation

and sport in which they can participate with the same degree of freedom as the able-bodied.'

People with 'problems', whether these are caused by defined mental illness or psychological imbalance as a result of stress (including disease) or trauma (accident or injury), may find especial satisfaction and enjoyment from swimming. The reason why they so benefit derives from a 'law of personal development levels' which works like this. Nature causes the functional organisms of a person with a 'problem' to regress down the scale of evolutionary development to a lower level where he is able to cope with the situation in which he finds himself in a state of natural balance. For example, he may revert to childish behaviour patterns where logic and reason are discarded and a more primitive emotional response takes over. Where bodily activity is concerned, this lower level becomes 'swimming level' where the person involved finds satisfaction and fulfilment in being balanced and supported in an environment similar to an embryonic state or an earlier evolutionary level. Many 'distressed' people therefore find they can cope in the supportive element of water in a way they are not able to on land; they may regain lost confidence or perhaps acquire it for the first time. Some of them may be able to transfer this confidence to other areas of life.

Nevertheless, to the nervous newcomer, especially if he or she suffers from a physical disability, a swimming pool in use by the general public may seem a particularly hostile environment. The noise and movement create an atmosphere of confusion and the floor around the pool looks slippery. Swimmers are thrashing about in all directions; others are diving or jumping in, and the danger of being bumped into or landed on may seem overwhelming. Childhood recollections may suggest that the water will only be a degree of two above freezing, that the steps will be difficult to negotiate (and they may well be!), that the changing-rooms will be crowded with hearty, shouting and obstreperously naked bodies and littered with misplaced socks and underwear, and that the showers, if they work, will be cold. To visualize the pool as a place of peace and quiet, a haven where body and spirit can be refreshed and re-created, may seem impossible.

It is true that it may sometimes be a mistake to introduce a disabled or handicapped non-swimmer to a pool when it is in busy general use. It is better to choose a time when the pool is reserved for disabled people or the age-group to which the individual belongs or, if this is not possible, to ask the manager to suggest a time when few people will be there. There may be a local swimming club catering specifically for disabled or handicapped people, with qualified teachers supported by several helpers and a weekly reservation of an hour or so for uninterrupted use of the pool. These clubs will organize galas and social events as well as swimming lessons and sessions, and help may be available with transport to and from the pool. Generally the clubs allow for most degrees and types of disability and membership costs very little. Membership of such a club does not detract from your independence and once you can swim with confidence you are free to join in the general public sessions if you want to. You should also find that the water is actually pleasantly warm, that the friendliness of your fellow members soon makes you feel secure and at home, and that the risk of accident is negligible.

Swimming has proved beneficial for people suffering from a very wide range of disabilities and handicaps. Indeed there are only a few contra-indications, apart from some merely temporary conditions. Those who are uncontrollably incontinent should not swim, nor those – in public anyway – with severe behavioural problems. Otherwise, the only people who should not swim are those who simply do not enjoy it. With some conditions (e.g. brittle bones) special precautions must be taken, but provided those responsible in the pool are fully aware of the condition and the precautions necessary then if the individual wants to swim he should be encouraged to do so.

What can disabled or handicapped people expect to gain from regular swimming? For some there may be a symptomatic improvement, especially for those rehabilitating after surgery. Exercise in the sustaining element of water helps to restore muscle function, for example, and strengthens connective tissues. This is perceived by doctors who recommend hydrotherapy to their patients as part of the recovery programme – a programme, incidentally, which all too often stops short the day the patient is discharged from hospital or at best is continued only for a few brief weekly or fortnightly sessions.

For many people, however, especially those with severe or multiple disabilities, or congenital conditions, or even those who consider themselves to be 'unfit' or 'below par' in an unspecified way, there would be little or no purpose in swimming for symptomatic improvement. If you have arthritis in your right arm, swimming purely to make your right arm 'better' could well be a waste of time. Medical science has conditioned us – most of us – to regard the body as a sort of machine made up of various components. If a component becomes faulty we visit our doctor for treatment, or our garage for a repair. If that does not solve the problem we are sent to a specialist in that component – let us say the rheumatologist. If the problem does not yield to his attentions we may be referred to the neurologist or the endocrinologist, and we may in time end up with the psychiatrist – or possibly with our dismissal and the words 'I'm sorry, you'll just have to live with it' ringing in our ears. Sometimes, of course, the machine concept works; a pill may be found for the particular ill or a surgeon may remove the malfunctioning part and leave us the better for its removal. Joint replacement therapy is one of the triumphs of this approach, certainly as far as older patients are concerned. But it is becoming more and more apparent that for certain conditions – cancer and multiple sclerosis among them – this mechanical model is not necessarily effective and different approaches are gaining adherents. The benefits of treating people instead of treating diseases are becoming obvious.

Swimming treats the whole person. It does so in a way which is impossible on land where gravity and hard surfaces intervene. The only equivalent, as astronauts have found, is in space where the body floats freely although as yet trammelled by protective clothing and equipment. What the disabled swimmer can expect, then, if he swims regularly and with some expenditure of energy, is a general overall physical improvement from a strengthening of tissues throughout the body, more effective blood circulation and a reduction in the normal heart rate. If the condition of the whole is improved then, unless there is some vital and irremediable severance, the condition of the part will improve also.

This is not all. Medical science, with its narrow concentration on specifics, often ignores or neglects the patient's state of mind. Yet without a positive mental approach recovery and rehabilitation will be delayed, or may never happen at all. The discipline of regular swimming – of regular exercise generally – demands a positive mental approach, a concentration on taking action oneself, not a dependence on action taken by others. Many disabled people feel themselves cut off from society by their disability, deterred from taking part in activities, sports and entertainments enjoyed by the able-bodied. If you are in a wheelchair, conversation tends to be carried on above your head with remarks and questions involving you being addressed to your companion – as summed up in the title of the BBC radio programme *Does he take sugar?* In a swimming pool, however, all heads are on the same level, and it is ability, not disability, that matters.

Looking at some of the more common handicaps and disabilities that afflict mankind, we shall find that it is the 'whole person benefit' gained from regular swimming that is the most significant corrective. In some instances measurable physical improvement may result after a few months; in others, there may be no apparent change in physical condition even after years. But it is quite misguided to assess the value of a therapy such as swimming in the same way that one might assess the efficacy of a course of medication. The stimulus, the enjoyment, the strengthening that comes from contact with others, the simple skills that may be slowly absorbed, the pride in achievement, the visual and spatial awareness, the benefits to the whole system from developing a regular pattern of breathing – these may be difficult or impossible to measure or quantify and cannot be subjected to the typical medico-scientific response of double-blind testing. Yet anyone involved in swimming therapy for any length of time will testify that they happen and make a contribution to the individual's quality of life that is of the highest value.

In recent years there have been radical changes in the ways that some conditions are treated. Most doctors now recognize that exercise is beneficial for asthma sufferers and the Institute of Swimming Teachers and Coaches has devised a programme of training and activity especially for them. There is also a National Asthma Swim Group Movement for children, which held the first of its National Galas in 1983. That asthma need be no handicap to performance is shown by the fact that in the 1976 Olympics five out of thirteen men and three out of fifteen women in the Australian swimming team either had asthma or had suffered from it in the past. The long-distance swimmer Alison Streeter has had asthma from infancy; in 1984 she swam the Channel for the fourth time, came second in the Catalina Channel race in California and became the first woman to swim around the Isle of Wight, covering 62 miles in twenty-one hours and easily breaking the previous record. The best known asthmatic swimmer is probably Dawn Fraser, who took up swimming 'to lick asthma' before its therapeutic effects were generally recognized and won gold medals in the Olympics in 1956, 1960 and 1964.

Swimming does not 'cure' asthma but it can greatly reduce its disabling effects. This is partly because any regularly undertaken physical exercise improves the body's efficiency generally. Asthma attacks become less frequent and less severe and the feeling of well-being after an exercise session helps to counteract the distress and depression often experienced. Swimming is especially valuable for those with exercise-induced asthma (EIA). This can be brought on by energetic exercise leading to the inhalation of large amounts of air with a comparatively low water vapour content. As the air inhaled by swimmers is especially humid they are far less likely to be affected by their exercise. The regular breathing needed for efficient swimming should also help to correct the aberrant habitual breathing pattern which is one of asthma's chief disabling effects.

Psychologically the benefits can be equally valuable. In the past, children with asthma tended to be protected from activity; they were fussed over, set apart, excused from games at school. The experience of the first of the children's swim groups, originating in 1978 in York as the result of initiatives by local doctors and involving a leading swimming coach, showed that as long as preventive medication was taken before the session began no problems occurred. The children gained in self-confidence, enjoyed themselves greatly, especially as water games were included in the programme, and benefited physically as well. The sessions also brought the parents together.

In succeeding years the Swim Group movement has spread throughout Britain with activity programmes being developed through paediatric units and galas at local and regional levels being organized, with Fison's Pharmaceuticals as major sponsors. Many children with asthma can lead full, happy and active lives without this type of structured programme, especially if their parents are positively advised and aware of the value of exercise. But it is clear that already there are thousands for whom the movement has proved extremely helpful and whose quality of life has been enhanced.

Adults benefit also from regular swimming, including those who have suffered from asthma for several decades. A recorded instance from a few years ago is that of Barry, a New Zealander of sixty-three, who took up swimming on his retirement to try to improve his condition. He built up to an hour's swimming a day, covering 1,500 metres, and walking or running as well. He succeeded in overcoming his long-standing pulmonary disability without having to use drugs and his swimming coach described his achievement as 'a new facet of thinking'.

Alan, who responded to the questionnaire, told of his own experience with chronic asthma. As a schoolboy he was an active sports enthusiast and after leaving school he took up manual work, keeping himself reasonably fit although asthma attacks occurred frequently. Then, aged twenty-six, he lost his job. 'I had to take up a sport,' he said, 'so that my breathing would not deteriorate.' He chose swimming mainly because it was convenient and cheap. 'My first dip was a real eye-opener,' he said. 'I could only swim two lengths before I had to stop – and I thought I was fit. Since that day I have slowly managed to work up until I could manage a total distance in one swim of 5½ miles.

Also since that day I have had only two slight asthma attacks. One was when the baths were shut for a month over Christmas and New Year and the other when I decided to give swimming a rest. Now I never swim less than 2½ miles a week and I have never felt so healthy and fit.'

Emily, now in her sixties, attests that she does not get exercise-induced asthma in the water. 'My asthma has got a lot better,' she says, 'but I'd dearly love to throw my inhalers away.' Emily is unhappy about the swimming facilities in her neighbourhood, however. 'It would be bliss for me if there were a special time when people swimming for health could have the pool to themselves. One of the sadnesses about Mrs Thatcher's rate policies is that some swimming pools have been closed. Brent used to have a very good, small, clean pool in Granville Road which has been closed, and I'm sure there are others. Too bad!'

It is estimated that about 8 million people in Great Britain suffer from one of the two hundred different forms of arthritic and rheumatic diseases. Osteoarthritis and rheumatoid arthritis are the commonest conditions. Recent research has led to great advances in joint replacement and safer and more effective drug treatment but, in the words of Dr C. Barnes, chairman of the Arthritis and Rheumatism Council's executive committee, 'there are many sufferers whose disease still progresses relentlessly towards disability and dependency.'

Exercise is generally recognized as a valuable therapy for people with rheumatic or arthritic conditions provided that it does not cause pain. However, often the exercise is confined to physiotherapy or hydrotherapy, with the patient being treated by someone else for short periods of time. No one suggests that regular swimming will produce a permanent cure but in many instances it proves extremely helpful in maintaining and/or restoring mobility. The support given by the water relieves pain and enables joints and muscles to be exercised weight-free in ways which would not be possible otherwise.

There is no need for age to be a deterrent. Margaret was nearly seventy before she learned to swim. Rheumatoid arthritis had been diagnosed some ten years previously. She was fitted with both hip and knee replacements and other joints were also affected. Her occupational therapist advised her to start swimming and encouraged her to join the local swimming club for handicapped people. There she was taught to swim and given a series of water exercises to ease her joints. 'I enjoy swimming and with rheumatoid arthritis it is the only exercise I can do with the minimum of pain,' she says. 'I am quite confident that it is only the swimming which keeps me mobile. At my age I feel privileged to be able to join and belong to the club.'

Mary was even older when she learned to swim. Suffering from arthritis in the knee, she began by visiting a hospital pool but, as she says, 'I waited till the age of seventy-three before accomplishing my heart's desire!' Like Margaret she joined a club affiliated to the Association of Swimming Therapy and she now swims once a week. Her arthritic condition may not have greatly improved but, she says, 'It has done a great deal for my mental attitude. I love going, and enjoy the company of very nice people and excellent teachers. Thank you!'

Dora, aged seventy, also has arthritis in the knee. By chance she heard a talk on the radio recommending swimming as a help to people with arthritis; otherwise no one had suggested it or given her any advice. She swims three times a week and has found that the pain is relieved and she can walk and sleep more easily. Her general health has also improved. Michael, in his late sixties, also gathered some hints about swimming from the media and now swims twice weekly, finding that it helps to control rheumatic pain and ease stiffness. 'It enables reasonable fitness and mobility to be maintained, with a good effect on muscles, heart, lungs and relaxation of mind and body,' he adds. Emily, in her sixties and with both arthritis and asthma, swims three times a week covering 1,000 metres each time, and claims increased mobility and a general feeling of being more fit. Muriel, sixty-four, also covers considerable distances, 600 metres generally five times a week. She lists four specific benefits: loosening of joints; less tendency to breathlessness on climbing stairs, doing heavy housework etc; very marked improvement in resistance to colds; and sound sleep. She took up swimming when arthritis in her knees made long-distance walking impossible. David, fifty, swims 400 metres twice a week to keep himself mobile. He has arthritis in the hips, lower back and neck. Doreen, likewise, swims twice weekly. 'I feel sure that had I not restarted swimming I would have stiffened up completely,' she says. 'I find it a most relaxing exercise, very helpful in muscle control and also good for one's breathing.' Gabriella, fifty-five, who has had both hips replaced, finds that her swimming has had a very considerable effect in aiding the movement of both legs and has also much improved her confidence.

Sometimes a very active life is seriously impeded or even brought to a complete standstill in middle age by an arthritic condition. Jo, in her fifties, leads such a life. She has chondro-calcinosis, a form of osteoarthritis, which has necessitated a series of operations on her knees and ankles. Swimming – up to twenty lengths two or three times a week – has been essential to keep her muscles in reasonable condition and to maintain a feeling of well-being and satisfaction from participating in a sporting activity.

An important point made by Jo and many others with arthritic and rheumatic conditions is that warm water, above 84°F, is necessary to keep them fully mobile. If the water is significantly cooler than this in your local pool where you swim regularly, you should discuss the temperature with the pool manager, who may be able to do something about it.

One of the commonest complaints that flesh – or rather the skeleton – is heir to is 'back trouble'. For all varieties of back problem swimming is effective therapy, but it is important to seek advice preferably from a physiotherapist, osteopath or a swim-oriented doctor about water exercise and choice of stroke. The majority of cases handled by osteopaths are concerned with back pain, whether deriving from poor posture, accident, 'wear and tear' or whatever, and swimming is very often recommended as exercise between treatments and then to prevent the problem recurring.

Alice, in her mid-forties, describes her experience in the simplest of terms. Suffering from back pain she began swimming twice weekly. Now, after two years, she says 'I feel very fit, free of pain and it helps to keep my weight down.' Maureen, fifty, reports in a little more detail: 'I have suffered from a bad back for eight years and should have started swimming before but always felt too exhausted after a busy day at work. Now my general health is better, I realize I must swim otherwise my spine will just go on getting stiffer. Swimming is the best exercise for me as I cannot hurt myself in water.' Judith, sixty-five, learnt to swim over twelve years ago when she was advised that it would help her back problem. She swims four times a week in winter and daily in summer, with a set of water exercises as well, following her osteopath's advice. She comments: 'Swimming has been indispensable in conjunction with osteopathic treatment to make me almost 100 per cent mobile. My osteopath has said my recovery has been mostly by my own efforts of swimming and exercise in water.'

Joanna, in her thirties, had pain and stiffness in the lumbar area and examination revealed several compressed discs. Both her physiotherapist and osteopath advised her to swim and she covers up to forty lengths three or four times a week, using both crawl and breaststroke. She says: 'At first I could only walk with pain, and swimming enabled me to regain movement in a natural manner since I did not have to avoid pain. Front crawl was the optimum stroke. I gained flexibility and overall increased fitness. Any pain I suffer now can be alleviated by a swim.' Susan, forty-eight, echoes Joanna's reference to a 'natural' manner. Having spent time in plaster for a disc problem, she rejected the offer of an operation and chose swimming instead, although neither her consultant nor general practitioner suggested it. Having been told that her spinal problem was the result of 'the wear and tear of years' – just natural use – she decided to use natural means to overcome the weakness. She swims almost every day, about thirty lengths, sometimes swimming with a friend 'as a good sociable activity, better than drinking coffee'. Regaining full fitness, she says, is 'a long, slow process, but I am almost able to lead a full and normal life again – except for sitting, which causes problems still. I know I will continue to swim because so much of one's body benefits from this natural flowing exercise.' Susan has developed a programme of water exercises for herself and has become a strong proponent of swimming as therapy. 'I suggest it as a remedy to anyone who "breathes" back problems. I also suggested a neurosurgeon friend in Canada might use it instead of the knife. "Pool's too cold," he said.'

The experiences of two elderly ladies are remarkable, not least for the courage and resourcefulness that both have shown. Marjorie, in her seventies, was diagnosed with a lesion in the lower four lumbar discs, resulting in temporary paralysis in her right leg. She has had hydrotherapy treatment in hospital and has been treated by an osteopath for the past seven years. She swims daily, if possible, about twenty lengths a time, using breast and backstroke, and has gained several Amateur Swimming Association Adult Awards. She joined a swimming club for disabled people and now teaches the non-swimmers. Swimming, she says, has had a tremendous effect on her efforts to regain and maintain health. 'I enter the pool often in pain but always feel eased of pain after a swim as well as a feeling of renewed energy and total relaxation physically and mentally.'

Kate, now eighty-three, also has a major back problem, badly damaged discs causing the vertebrae to shift easily, resulting in considerable pain. She spends much of the day lying down. About seven years ago Kate was advised by her doctor to swim on her back as frequently as she could and she now swims about 250 metres five times a week. Swimming is the only exercise that does not aggravate her condition and has helped her develop the muscles in her back to some extent. But it has done more for Kate than this. 'Swimming has been very morale boosting for me. It is the only time of day when I feel normal. By strengthening the back muscles I can be up a little longer and do a little more about the house (though I am essentially bedridden and have frequent relapses). Without swimming I would be completely helpless by now.' Kate has obtained one Amateur Swimming Association Diamond Award and one Gold and is on her way to a second Gold – an extraordinary achievement, which her husband, who transports her to and from the pool and is always on hand while she is swimming, must be proud to share.

Lastly, Penny may stand as representative of the many people whose back problem would force them out of work were it not for the relief afforded by swimming. Now in her mid-forties, about three years ago she suffered two slipped discs, causing chronic stiffness and immobility of the spine. She turned to swimming of her own volition, visiting the pool as often as possible and swimming up to twenty-five lengths each time. The results she expresses quite simply: 'Without swimming I feel that I would not have overcome the problems of a weak spine. I should not be able to carry on with my job as Sister of an Intensive Care Unit.'

Other orthopaedic problems can be resolved or at least aided by swimming. Mary, sixty-eight, injured her shoulders, possibly as a result of heavy lifting when nursing in younger days. She swims several lengths every weekday and claims, 'If it wasn't for my swimming and simple daily exercises I am sure my arms, neck and shoulders would have seized up completely. I feel relaxed and invigorated.' Alfred, who is about the same age, had knee trouble as well as being overweight. A friend, who was using swimming as therapy for his back, suggested that he try it and he set out on a twice weekly programme, up to forty lengths each time. His knees recovered and he lost nearly two stone in weight. Alfred is a sheet metal worker, still working a five-and-a-half day week. 'I feel that people of my age should find all the exercise they need to keep fit by swimming,' he comments. 'You do it as slow or fast as you care to but all the time you are using more muscles than any form of exercise I know.'

Both Jean and Amanda are members of the same

swimming club for disabled people. Jean, fifty-four, was born with fixed hips, and other joints eventually began to stiffen. She sought medical advice and felt that the only suggestion worth following up was to learn how to swim. It took nearly two years before she began to feel any benefit and she now reports that there has been a small improvement in her hips and other joints although stiffness is still apparent at times. Her muscle tone and general health have improved. Jean has won several medals in galas at all levels. Amanda, nineteen, is one of the youngest members of the club. Her knees dislocate easily and swimming is the only exercise open to her. Luckily she has always enjoyed it. 'Swimming has not only improved my health generally but also strengthened my leg muscles. This has been a great help in controlling my knees,' she says. Amanda continues, 'Swimming gives many people, much more disabled than myself, a feeling of self-confidence as well as something to strive for. People who have no use in their legs are given a buoyancy in the water which makes them independent. I look forward to Monday nights at the pool and I think that it is very important to have a special session for disabled swimmers in every town.'

Until recently little was done to help rehabilitate the victims of major multiple handicapping diseases, many of whom were left to moulder away in wheelchair or bed with the focus only on everything they were unable to do. With the growth of voluntary societies seeking to give a voice to disabled people and their relatives, and with a more positive approach to disability in general, the situation is rapidly changing. Cerebral palsy affects between twenty and twenty-five children in every 10,000, damaging the central nervous system and usually causing spasticity, athetosis or paralysis of one or more limbs. Speech and other senses may also be impaired. Swimming is valuable here as it helps to inculcate skills and to produce a sense of achievement with a heightening of self-respect. It is enjoyable and may also be competitive for even the most seriously affected, as for purposes of swimming competition the degrees of disability have been divided into eight categories from quadraplegic to minimally affected. Competition takes place up to Olympic and World Championship standards; in the 1985 Cerebral Palsy Olympics, held in Austria, Britain entered the smallest team of only six swimmers who came back with nineteen medals, nine of them gold.

Symptomatic improvement is not likely to occur with cerebral palsy swimmers, although Martin, whose story is told in Chapter 6, has noted some improvement. Val, thirty-four, makes the strongest argument for its therapeutic value. She has been swimming for about twenty years, up to twelve lengths a time, mostly on her back, often using a flotation suit to keep her afloat when training. Unlike many cerebral palsy swimmers who are members of special clubs Val prefers to work things out on her own and competes in galas up to international level. She makes it clear that she swims for the pleasure of it. 'Although I am unable to walk, I crawl about my flat which, I feel, gives me all the exercise I need. I swim because I enjoy it. I recommend swimming to everyone, disabled and able-bodied, as a form of relaxation and as a very good way of meeting people.' In the 1986 International Cerebral Palsy Games in Belgium, Val won two gold medals in her class, both in world record time.

It is estimated that about 50,000 people in Britain have multiple sclerosis, a disease that also damages the central nervous system and may cause progressive paralysis and impairment of the senses. Controlled breathing, relaxation, diet and exercise are at least as effective in managing the condition as costly hospital treatment. Many multiple sclerosis sufferers find they can move far more fluently and easily in water than they can on land, and swimming, provided that over-exertion is avoided, is again valuable therapy.

Both Anne and Isabel are confined to wheelchairs for most of their day. Anne, thirty-four, began swimming as a means of maintaining her strength and built up rapidly to sixteen lengths a day, four or five times a week. She feels, she says, 'much "better" afterwards' and it helps to relieve soreness in her back. Isabel, forty-five, has been swimming for more than ten years, going two or three times a week, swimming about four lengths and working through various water exercises. 'I am much better if I go,' she says. 'For a while I only swam once a week and I could only manage half a length. I will try and never get to that state again!' It is sad to note that neither Anne nor Isabel had swimming suggested to them by their doctors.

Since the use of the vaccine has become widespread poliomyelitis occurs only rarely in Britain but there are still many people who have been disabled by the disease in earlier years. Pat, in her mid-forties, has been left with severely weakened legs and left shoulder and uses a wheelchair. She began regular swimming after a seaside holiday and tries to swim on her front to improve her breathing. After less than a year she noted that her thigh and upper arm muscles were streng-thening. She defines other benefits: 'It is very nice to participate in a sport with the family and not either sit on the side line or participate only with disabled people. The staff at the pool are very helpful and I have been able to take my eight year old son swimming whenever I wish – and of course swim myself.'

A full and eloquent account comes from another polio victim, Ann, now in her seventies. She contracted the disease in infancy and was left lame in her right leg. She wore a calliper until she was fifteen; then she underwent an arthrodesis operation to fix her ankle immovably. Now she has a stiff ankle, a moderately straight leg 2½ inches short, and a double curvature of the spine. She writes:

> Although my disability was comparatively slight, I have never run, jumped, skipped or danced – walking was always a chore rather than a pleasure. I have, however, lived a very normal life until at the age of forty-eight I slipped and fractured the tibia in my lame leg. This resulted in a long period of incapacity – nearly two years – resulting in much weakness of both legs. The bone did not start to heal for nearly a year.
>
> Once again mobile, I started to take swimming lessons – I could always float and play around in the water but had never learned to control my movements. In learning this I found that I was using muscles in the right leg which I had never used before, and this I find amazing. One is told that muscles atrophy without use, but after nearly fifty years my muscles responded gradually and I am now able to control my leg better than I ever did when I was more mobile. In learning to balance my body in the water I found it much easier to control my stance out of it, and my legs are stronger now than they ever were.
>
> So much for the physical side – but psychologically it has been an even greater boost. To be able to move easily and gracefully, to stand on my right leg only without aid in the water, and in many other ways to enjoy physical effort with some success has really given me a new enjoyment of life. Also I am lucky in that my body formation is such that I float without effort vertically as well as on my back, and I have been able to instill confidence into people who are physically fitter and much younger than myself. To be able to help others is a grand tonic!

Another moving account comes from Paul, thirty-one, who was born with spina bifida. This necessitated a series of major operations and these, with the effects of the disease itself, have resulted in severe impairment of balance and mobility. Paul learned to swim as a child; now he swims three times a week, covering 4,000 metres each session – 160 lengths of the normal pool. He summarizes his experience:

> Swimming has allowed me to take safe and proper exercise as no other sport can. The risk of cuts, knocks or broken bones is diminished and my lack of balance compensated for. Through swimming I have been able to gain confidence, strength and, above all, enjoyment, all of which promote health and happiness.
>
> In 1984 I had the honour of representing Great Britain in the British Paralympic Swimming Team for the VII World Wheelchair Games at Stoke Mandeville. This was an exhilarating experience, not only for the pleasure of competing but the joy of seeing disabled people liberated from the confines of wheelchairs and walking aids and able to express their prowess on equal terms with able-bodied people.
>
> In the future I hope to concentrate more on coaching than competing and so give something back to the sport I've gained so much from.

The largest group of people who benefit from swimming – a group to which very many of us belong at one time or another – consists of those who are recovering from accident, injury, operation or trauma such as a heart attack. Unless swimming is medically contra-indicated it can help greatly in rehabilitation. There are obvious physical benefits: stimulus to joints and muscles, being able to exercise in a weight-free condition, improvement to circulation and heart action. Confidence may be restored and a sense of well-being regained. The positive and regular breathing necessary for efficient swimming is an important factor in achieving full response and recovery of mind and body. A hydrotherapy pool is standard equipment in most major hospitals as a recognized aid to rehabilitation. But these pools are small, the demands on them are high and they are labour-intensive. Treatment normally ends with discharge from hospital. What all major hospitals need is a warm, 15-metre pool for the use of both in- and out-patients, supervised by physiotherapists who are also trained swimming teachers. This would be of greater benefit to more people than the vastly expensive complex items of diagnostic and physiotherapy equipment now in fashion, with the demands they make on limited budgets and charitable giving and the distancing of the human element in care and treatment.

Veronica, fifty-two, argues a strong case. She was involved in a serious motor accident in which both her feet were fractured. She was confined to bed in hospital for six weeks and, following discussion with her consultant and physiotherapist, began swimming soon after discharge. She swims three times a week, when possible, up to twenty lengths each time. 'I was pleasantly surprised that I could swim eight lengths the first time I went, but slowly and with a rest after each length. Fitness improved rapidly, both in general terms and in the mobility of the feet. By the end of the summer vacation I had improved greatly and was feeling reasonably fit.'

Her hospital experience, Veronica found, was disenchanting. 'I felt far too little attention was paid to fitness both in hospital and for out-patients. If I had eaten half the food offered I would have gained weight and found it harder to walk again. I also think I should have had far more effective physiotherapy, and swimming is the obvious exercise for anyone with foot injuries if they are not encumbered with dressings. I have recently attended weekly classes with a teacher of Alexander Technique which has benefited me even more. While my orthopaedic consultant seemed to accept that I should have to put up with a limp and reduced mobility, my Alexander teacher has taught me to walk pretty normally.'

Christina, in her sixties, also suffered a leg injury in a road accident and subsequently had to have a leg amputated. She swims twice a week and although she covers only short distances she finds it keeps her muscles supple and that she enjoys it. Phyllis, in her mid-seventies, fractured the neck of a femur in an accident and had to have a hip replacement. She ascribes her speedy recovery to the fact that she was swimming daily until just before the accident, and it has helped to restore muscle tone since.

Mike, in his early fifties, was another road accident victim. This happened when he was twenty-eight; his right leg had to be amputated and his left leg suffered multiple fractures. He spent several months in hospital under traction, followed by several more months of physiotherapy. Mike had been a keen sportsman but, he says, 'I thought at the time "that's it – I'm finished at the age of twenty-eight".' When a physiotherapist suggested he try swimming Mike at first was terrified at the idea. Eventually he began, and later the birth of a daughter who loved the water from an early age encouraged him to increase his involvement. He qualified as a club instructor and then as a swimming teacher. 'I now swim more than ever before,' he says, 'despite arthritis in my arms and hands, which doesn't bother me as it does some people. I am convinced beyond any shadow of doubt that swimming has pulled me through the bad times and certainly made the good times better.'

Recently Mike completed a 2-mile inshore swim, for which he was awarded a trophy. He trained for this by swimming sixty lengths three times a week. With little use in his remaining leg he depends almost entirely on arm movements, and like some other arm-only swimmers he can manage a good turn of speed. Mike's 2-mile swim was sponsored and raised about £500 for the British Legion Poppy Fund.

John, sixty-two, used swimming to help him recover strength and fitness after a heart attack and now feels fitter than ever. Emma was in the pool soon after a hysterectomy, swimming thirty-six lengths twice a week. Alan, fifty-seven, was advised by his osteopath to swim to help free a trapped nerve and built up to a hundred lengths a day, every day. He appreciates it as a non-violent form of exercise and a speedy way of recovering fitness. Mary, sixty, and Barbara, in her forties, both swim to improve mobility and flexibility after suffering strokes. Juliette, eighteen, learned to swim after being dropped into the pool at the age of six months. She injured her back in a riding accident and now swims for the therapeutic benefits and is also a member of a life-saving club. Richard, thirty-eight, was swimming within three weeks of a bilateral inguinal hernia operation, covering thirty to forty lengths most days of the week. Claire, twenty-three, a physiotherapist, suffered persistently from both glandular fever and asthma in her late teens. She took up swimming to help with breathing difficulties and now swims up to 150 lengths a time. Her own physical improvements so impressed her that she joined the Swimming Teachers' Association and is now involved with teaching swimming to disabled people.

Loss or severe impairment of one or more senses need not be an impediment to swimming. Mark, age twelve and partially blind, recommends swimming as an ideal sport for partially sighted children and himself swims nine lengths twice a week. Neil, totally blind, competes regularly in galas, swimming on his back and using the lane divider as a guide. Blind swimmers need auditory signals from the pool side to warn them when to turn, and deaf swimmers need visual signals from time to time or, when competing, to be tapped on the shoulder to know when to start. National and international competitions are organized for both deaf and blind swimmers and they also take part in galas for disabled swimmers generally.

Among the most severe of handicaps is the combination of deafness and blindness. The deaf-blind child lives in a world where objects for the most part are hostile and where movement is perilous and often painful. In the medium of water, however, the deaf-blind child or adult can move freely with far less risk of harm or hurt. The value of the swimming pool as a medium of instruction, another way through to the less able students, is recognized by SENSE, the National Deaf-Blind and Rubella Association, which has recently built a pool at its residential home for young adults. The Principal of the home outlines the value of the pool in three particular areas:

> to develop muscular control with those students who show need;
> to develop personal relationships between students and care-givers, sharing the water and inevitably coming into physical contact;
> to use the medium of warm water to relax the body and hopefully free it of twitches and other distractions, so enhancing the ability to attend with meaning.

Many physically disabled swimmers speak of the psychological benefits they have gained. Similar benefits accrue to the able-bodied. Edna, for example, in her late seventies, has been swimming three or four times a week for seven years and finds that her mental reactions are sharper. She can also walk and cycle longer distances. Christopher, thirty-eight, began swimming to improve fitness but found an unexpected but at least equally important psychological bonus. 'The break at lunchtime was very good for me. It cleared the mind and I was ready to start work again.' Robin, thirty, swam back into shape after having a baby and continues to average ninety lengths several times a week as she believes it keeps her healthier, less likely to contract disease and also 'much better emotionally'. Christine, forty-six, finds she has more energy for everyday living: 'My brain is able to retain important data. It makes me a more efficient person both at work and at home. Breathing is far easier.' Rosemary, sixty, says that her regular swimming provides relaxation and considerably reduces nervous tension. For Lorna, sixty-three, it helps to maintain a balanced outlook on life, while it has given Maureen, forty-eight, more confidence in herself. She tries, she says, 'to use the water as a friendly medium, not to fight against it'. Fred, fifty-three, who was born with a speech defect, took up swimming in an attempt to improve his confidence in himself. The only professional advice he has received, he says, is to 'just keep swimming'. He finds that his ability in the water helps him to deal with the problems of everyday life. Chris, forty-two, enjoys 'helpful chatter in the pool and changing room with very friendly encouraging people'. Marjorie, in her seventies, is one of many who talk of the 'total relaxation, physically and mentally' that she obtains from the pool. Several people describe swimming as a form of meditation, while Linda, an excellent and stylish swimmer, takes this further: 'When you feel you are useless or worthless, to go and do something *well* gives quite a lift to the spirits. Also it's like meditation. You are in your own world and no one can reach you. I suppose it's my form of relaxation. And what I find interesting is that on the days I least want to go I usually swim best.' Emma, seventy, who has been swimming only since she retired five years ago and now swims almost every day up to sixty-six lengths a time, sums up in two succinct sentences: 'I think people who go to psychiatrists would do better to swim. Exercise eliminates stress.' Finally Olga, sixty-one, herself a doctor, tries to swim three or four times a week because, she says, 'it keeps me healthy and energetic, able to cope with an exacting and demanding profession.'

What is common to all who have written or spoken about their experiences with swimming is their optimism and spirit. There is criticism of facilities, organization and sometimes of the lack of advice and encouragement but at the same time there is genuine appreciation of the opportunities that are available and of the help given by teachers and instructors. The determination shown by many disabled swimmers is often remarkable. Many swim several times a week, but this involves not merely swimming but getting to the pool, negotiating the building and changing rooms, possibly in a wheelchair or with crutches or walking frame, undressing, entering and leaving the water – often made needlessly difficult by poorly designed steps – showering, dressing and so on.

In answer to the question 'What help or advice have you had in your pursuit of better health through swimming?' about half our swimmers replied 'None'. Of the rest, several received encouragement from friends, a few had been advised to swim by an osteopath or physiotherapist, and fewer still by a doctor. In some areas doctors do work closely with the local swimming club for handicapped people but many disabled swimmers do not wish to, or feel they do not need to, join a special club. About a quarter of our swimmers belong to a special club; the others use a public pool either in general time or in protected sessions, while some have the use of private pools belonging to sports clubs or other organizations. Whatever pool they use, however, there is no doubt that many, if not most, disabled swimmers do have to manage without much in the way of help, advice or training. What is even more significant is that there must be thousands of disabled people who would benefit from swimming and yet are completely unaware that this might be so.

The argument can be reinforced by considering a further three examples of disabled swimmers, all quite young. David, thirty-four, is blind and also has Still's disease, a severe form of rheumatoid arthritis. He swims up to fifteen lengths once a week to benefit his health. Sarah, twenty-eight, is poorly sighted and has cystic fibrosis – until lately it was very unusual for anyone with this disease to survive into adulthood. She swims as often as she can (she is in fact a doctor so the opportunities are limited) as an activity she can enjoy with others and to build up her strength. Joan, thirty-three, had a brain tumour and after surgery suffered a left hemiparesis – a partial paralysis of the left side of the body. She has also had Addison's disease and a papilloma cancer. She swims for two hours once a week. 'It has maintained what use I have left,' Joan says. 'It has helped sharing with others and making sure that once a week all my family get involved. It builds up confidence and helps one to recover more quickly from setbacks.' If David, Sarah and Joan can benefit from swimming then, one might think, there cannot be many, no matter what their condition, who would not similarly benefit.

There are two groups of people about whom particular questions regarding the advisability of swimming have been raised: those with epilepsy, and the mentally impaired. Over the years there has been much debate about whether people with epilepsy should swim. It does seem that the possible perils have been greatly exaggerated and that the over-protective attitudes have been based on needless apprehension. The lives of those with epilepsy are restricted enough as it is and swimming gives them an enjoyable activity of much social and psychological benefit.

However, it is essential that anyone with epilepsy, or the parents of younger children suffering from it, should consult the family doctor to ascertain that there is nothing in the person's condition that might be triggered off by the pool environment. If the 'all clear' is given and swimming is approved then there should be no special problem provided certain measures are taken.

The pool manager should be told that the swimmer has epilepsy; difficulties are far more likely to arise if the condition is not disclosed. The swimmer should be accompanied by a companion who is a competent swimmer, who can recognize an attack if it occurs and knows what to do. This applies to all types of fit or seizure, but usually action is only needed in the case of major seizure or *grand mal*. The seizure itself is not dangerous and there is less chance of harm to the individual in water than there is on land, provided the head is kept clear of the water and supported throughout the attack. Someone on the pool side should also observe the swimmer and be ready to go for help if an emergency occurs. It is best to avoid periods when the pool is likely to be crowded and if there is a local swimming club for handicapped or disabled people it may be worth considering joining it.

It is the wary social attitude towards epilepsy that has caused most of the problems, by making sufferers reluctant to reveal their condition. They have either avoided swimming altogether or have swum keeping their condition secret, with at times troublesome consequences. Pool managers nowadays are ready to welcome swimmers with epilepsy provided that they are properly accompanied and the situation is understood.

As long as the same sort of precautions are taken, people with epilepsy should also be able to swim within their depth in the calm sea.

Mental impairment should not be a barrier to swimming. In this regard, the story of Doran, widely known through the book *Doran: Child of Courage* by his mother Linda Scotson, and through television, is inspirational. Born with severe brain damage, Doran was unable to see, hear or speak and was unable to co-ordinate his limbs. Mrs Scotson, whose husband had died before Doran was born, refused to accept the verdict of the medical establishment that there were at best only minimal prospects of improvement in her son's condition, and she took him against advice to the Institute for the Achievement of Human Potential in Philadelphia. Following their instructions she adapted her home, recruited a team of hard-working and dedicated volunteers, and worked with Doran intensively and unremittingly, seeking to give him a full range of controlled movement and to develop complete response in all his senses. Readers of the book, and those who have seen the television programmes, can judge her success for themselves.

In the early months of Doran's life, however, and before she had experienced the full range of doctors and their gloomy prognoses, Mrs Scotson came to realize that Doran needed a daily experience that would make his life worth living. Instinctively she chose swimming, although the nearest pool was 13 miles away and she had little money to spare for petrol and entrance charges. Every day, week after week, she took Doran and her four-year-old daughter Lili to the pool. They swam for an hour in the morning and an hour after eating a picnic lunch. Doran loved it. Other mothers regarded him as a two-month-old baby with defective eyesight; in fact he was seven months old, unable to control his eyes or movements, his muscles stiff, his movements spastic.

Desperately short of money, Mrs Scotson used funds set aside for the electricity bill to pay for the visits to the pool. She received no help from the Department of Health and Social Security, but the situation was saved by a considerate charity and by the pool management who gave her free entry when it was understood why she came so often. The swimming continued regularly.

A series of medical examinations and consultations at about this time seemed to show that there was no hope of significant progress. Nevertheless, in Mrs Scotson's words, 'The swimming had changed Doran. He was communicating with people. He smiled more than he cried. He ceased to cry the moment his request was granted.' Despite medical opinion this gave her encouragement and hope and she continued with the swimming practice until Doran was accepted for assessment and treatment in Philadelphia. From then on it was a different story.

Swimming for the mentally impaired may simply provide a welcome opportunity for fun in a comparatively safe setting. Or the swimming may be part of a larger programme designed to help the individual make the best use of his abilities. Such programmes are dependent on the level of understanding and degree of co-ordination and motor ability of the individual, and the teaching itself demands patience and the ability to break down each skill into a series of simple steps. In a hospital or residential home the swimming, or water activity, should be part of a coherent training programme. Teaching is through a variety of games and activities each of which has a specific objective: to develop awareness of different parts of the body, to practise symmetrical and alternating movements, to improve concentration, to co-ordinate the use of eyes and hands, and so on. Progressive training helps to build up confidence and skills. Beginning with adjustment to water, a programme might proceed through movements, activities and games, using various aids and items of equipment and, at times, music, and on to swimming strokes, independent swimming and simple life-saving exercises. The more enjoyable and stimulating the programme, the more successful it is likely to be.

For the mentally impaired, both adults and children, the pool should be a valuable learning centre. The Yorktown teaching pool in Arlington, Virginia, has the letters of the alphabet, various coloured geometrical designs, the cardinal compass points, the numbers 1–9 and the four basic arithmetical symbols on the tiled pool floor as well as animal and fish pictures on the walls. Colour coding to indicate depth and exits from the pool is another means of learning reinforcement. A sound system through which music could be broadcast underwater and the use of coloured lighting of differing intensity – provided that no troublesome reflections are cast on the water surface – would complete what might prove an ideal specification for a learning environment.

Children with Down's syndrome – Mongolism as it used to be known – especially seem to enjoy swimming. Many are keen competitors and delight enormously in any success they may achieve as well as greatly enjoying simply taking part. They also benefit from improvement in their breathing pattern which, as recent evidence suggests, is complemented by improvement in their mental capacity.

With these children, as with all children and adults who are mentally impaired or retarded from whatever cause or reason, the worst thing to do is to categorize them and then treat them according to what may be expected. This is where it can all go wrong. The teacher loses patience because the learner does not come up to expectations; the learner becomes frustrated because he cannot comprehend what is expected of him and he may express that frustration by aggressive or unco-operative behaviour. For the teacher the method should be to play to strengths not to weaknesses, to abilities not to disabilities, never to jump to conclusions and never to underestimate.

Those who are mentally impaired may also have physical disabilities and be in poor condition. One of the advantages of swimming as a therapy is that the disabilities may be less marked or troublesome in water than on land and the exercise may gradually help to improve the physical condition by strengthening the muscles and connective tissues, stimulating the circulation and increasing the lung capacity. Great care may be needed in handling the swimmers but the physical contact in itself can prove especially beneficial.

Generally speaking, it is inadvisable for mentally impaired swimmers, apart from young children, to use the pool in public sessions when they are liable to be confused and distracted by the noise and movement around them.

4

Into Action

If you are handicapped or disabled in some way – or the caring relative of someone who is – or if you are recuperating after a spell in hospital or recovering from an accident or injury, what should you do if swimming as a therapy appeals to you?

Much depends upon your own mobility. If you can walk unaided, can see and hear moderately well, have no serious problem with balance, are not subject to fits, and are sufficiently agile to get in and out of the pool without help (bearing in mind that the steps may be poorly designed), then there is probably no reason why you should not manage perfectly well at a general session in a public pool. Unless you are already a competent swimmer it is best to go with a friend, certainly for the first few visits. You do not necessarily need your doctor's blessing but if he knows about swimming he may be able to advise on strokes, techniques or any water exercises that may help. A physiotherapist or osteopath would probably be able to help you, and you may also benefit from a session of two with a swimming coach or teacher.

If your mobility, hearing or sight, balance or agility are much impaired, however, you may need to swim as a member of a special club. Action then takes place as follows:

1. See your general practitioner, hospital doctor or other therapist who is primarily responsible for your treatment and say that you want to swim regularly. You will need a medical note to join a special club and you may have to sign a disclaimer to protect the club from liability.

2. Discover from the local swimming pool, social services department, reference library or other likely source the name and address of the organizer of any swimming club for disabled people in your area. The National Association of Swimming Clubs for the Handicapped (NASCH) publishes a register of these clubs.

3. Contact the organizer and explain the nature of your disability or illness. You will probably have to complete a form with the relevant information. Join the next club session at the pool.

In areas where there are no special clubs the swimming pools usually have protected sessions for specified age groups or for 'disabled swimmers'. Investigate beforehand to see if one of these sessions may be suitable for you.

Most of the clubs operate under the umbrella of one of the nationwide organizations which have been established in recent years. These organizations, together with the Amateur Swimming Association, the Swimming Teachers' Association, the Royal Life Saving Society and other societies and associations with similar concerns, are members of the Sports Council's National Co-ordinating Committee on Swimming for the Disabled. This committee publishes a series of helpful booklets dealing with many aspects of the subject which is available from the member associations. The Amateur Swimming Association and the Swimming Teachers' Association run courses for teachers of disabled swimmers.

The three organizations primarily concerned with swimming for disabled people are the British Sports Association for the Disabled (BSAD), the Association of Swimming Therapy (AST), and NASCH. Founded in 1961, BSAD is recognized by the Sports Council as the body primarily responsible for the co-ordination and development of sport for disabled people. It operates through a network of clubs, centres, colleges and schools and covers a wide range of disability groups. Like other organizations BSAD runs competitive galas both for specific disability groups and for swimmers with a variety of handicaps.

The Association of Swimming Therapy was founded by James McMillan in 1950 with twelve disabled girls from the Halliwick School, Southgate. It uses its own teaching system called the Halliwick method and trains its own instructors. About ninety clubs are now affiliated to the AST with a regional organization, and national and regional galas and proficiency tests for swimmers and non-swimmers are organized. The Halliwick method is based on principles of hydromechanics and body mechanics. To begin with, teaching is on a one-to-one basis and no artificial aids, such as armbands or floats, are used. Swimmers are taught to adjust to water and to accept and make use of its power. They learn how to rotate and control their body movements in water and eventually how to move independently using a modified form of back crawl. The Halliwick method may be most suitable for the more severely mentally and physically handicapped.

The National Association of Swimming Clubs for the Handicapped has a large number of affiliated clubs, trains teachers and issues badges of endeavour to disabled swimmers. Galas also feature in its projects. NASCH recognizes that the best policy for disabled people in general is integration rather than segregation, but it is also aware that 'one reason why special clubs are popular with physically handicapped people is that they do not always feel like "appearing in public" in swimsuits'.

There are also clubs or organized sessions for people with particular disabilities. Branches of the Multiple Sclerosis Society, for example, may hold swimming sessions, as do Mencap and other voluntary organizations. In Bath there are sessions reserved for those disabled by polio and for those with arthritis and rheumatism, while Bristol has time set aside for back pain sufferers and for the visually handicapped. In some towns the swimming club is a section of a larger sports club for disabled people, or the local 'able-bodied' swimming club may run a section for disabled swimmers. In all there are about 300 special swimming clubs in the United Kingdom; in addition, many elderly disabled people attend sessions reserved for the 'over-sixties' or 'senior citizens'.

The number of different organizations involved may seem confusing and wasteful of resources but this is not necessarily so. Each organization sees itself as fulfilling a particular need and it develops its own methods and approach. The newly formed club, or the individual, therefore has a choice. It is important to explore the alternatives. For example, the AST's Halliwick method eschews the use of artificial aids, relying solely on the hands of the helper. Yet the ASA's paper on *The Principles of Teaching* says that 'the advantages of buoyancy aids can outweigh any disadvantages'. The club or individual has to decide which course to follow. Although the organizations may not always speak in harmony, it is best to regard them as complementary to each other or as alternatives rather than as rivals. There is no one correct method of teaching a disabled person to swim; the method chosen must suit the individual, not the other way around.

In many areas, however, there are no special swimming clubs. Not only that: there may be no swimming pool for many miles. In this situation things become more difficult but it does not mean that it should be impossible, except perhaps in the remotest parts of the countryside, for disabled people to enjoy the therapeutic benefits of swimming.

Anyone can start a swimming club for handicapped people providing that the will and energy are there. A tried and tested method exists for doing this, based on the experience of one of the oldest and most successful clubs, the Kensington Emperors. To follow this, let us assume that you are a relative or friend of a seriously disabled person. You have heard of the benefits that other disabled people have obtained from swimming and your doctor has confirmed that this would be 'a good idea'. So, what do you do?

1. Recruit two or three people to help you – relatives or friends of other disabled people and/or people that you know have an interest in swimming. Include someone who is disabled, if possible. Contact the organizers of the nearest special club (use the NASCH Register or phone the swimming pool for information) and arrange to visit them and learn as much as you can about the way they work and the problems they have faced and overcome.

2. Visit the swimming pool and discuss your project with the manager. The nearest public pool, because of distance, inadequate

facilities for disabled people or other reasons, may not be your choice. Alternatives are school pools, pools belonging to social clubs or large firms, even hospital pools. It is important that the water can be heated to 84–89°F and that access for wheelchairs is possible. Your club will need exclusive use of the pool and changing rooms at least once a week for at least one hour. Make sure that qualified life-saving cover will be available.

3. Discuss your project with the District Community Physician, local doctors that may be interested and sympathetic, the local hospital social worker and the Director of Social Services for your locality. Consult the nearest branch of the Red Cross and St John's Ambulance and seek their co-operation. Local branches of societies for handicapped people – the Multiple Sclerosis Society, the Arthritis & Rheumatism Council, for instance – may be interested and willing to help. Organizations involved in community service, including youth clubs, colleges and secondary schools, may be able to offer pool-side and changing room assistance. Exchange ideas with the officers of any local swimming club – perhaps your club could operate as a section of theirs, which might be an ideal arrangement.

4. Finance, especially at the outset, may be needed. Aim to get the interest and support of local business organizations such as Rotary, Round Table or Lions. Transport is often a problem and you may need to hire a

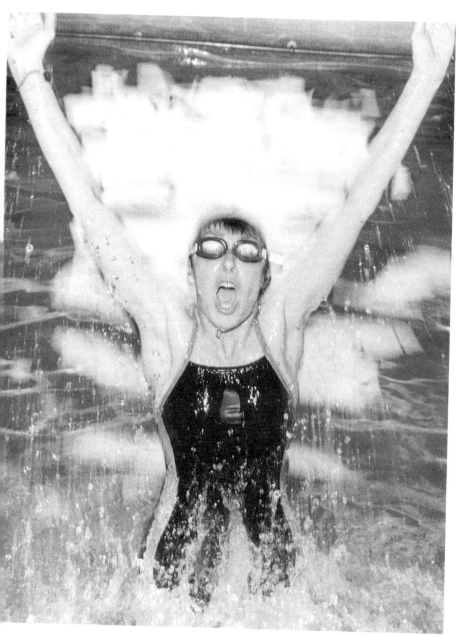

Into action.

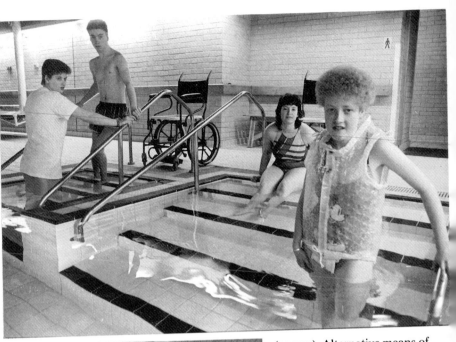

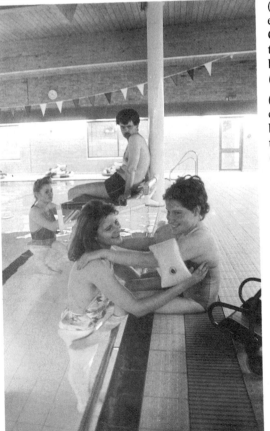

(ABOVE). Alternative means of entry to the National Star Centre pool. The swimmer in the foreground is wearing a bubble jacket flotation aid. (*National Star Centre*)

(LEFT). Into the pool. The correct way to lift. In the background a swimmer is using the electrically operated hoist. (*National Star Centre*)

(OPPOSITE ABOVE). Further means of entry/exit at the National Star Centre. Note the asymmetrical handrails, and the ease of access i a deck level pool. (*National Star Centre*)

(OPPOSITE BELOW). Entering the water using the hoist at the Lord Butler Leisure Centre, Saffron Walden. This member of the St Christopher Club is wearing a bubble jacket.

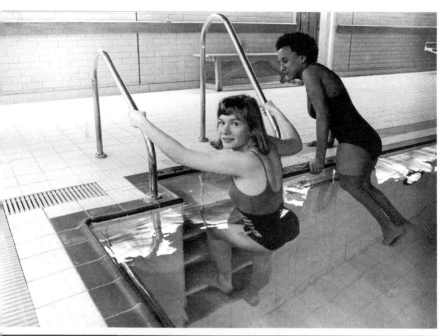

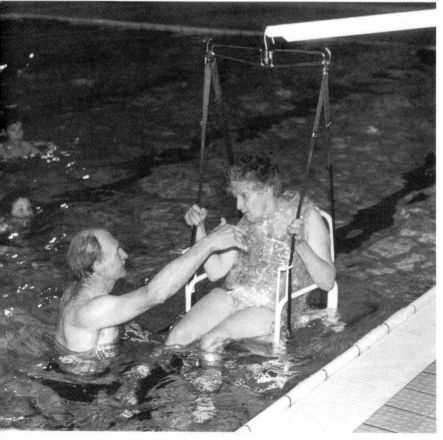

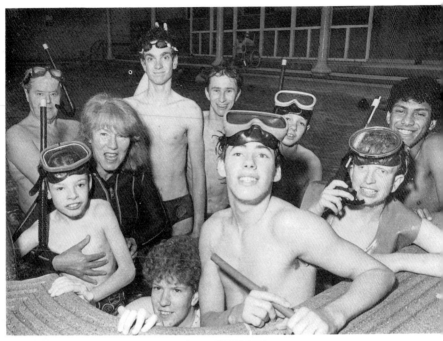

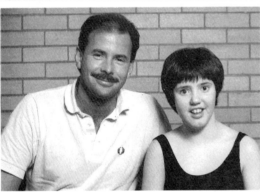

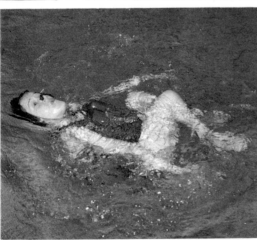

(ABOVE). Jill Myers (Chapter 4) and members of the Guillemot Branch of the British Sub-Aqua Club.

(LEFT TOP). Clare, a young swimmer with the St Christopher Club, with Olympic gold medallist David Wilkie. (*St Christopher Club*)

(LEFT BOTTOM). Val (Chapter 3) Gold Medal winner at the International Cerebral Palsy Games, 1986.

(OPPOSITE ABOVE). The new Kingfisher Pool at Sudbury.

(OPPOSITE CENTRE). The competition pool at the Crown Pools complex, Ipswich. (*Ipswich District Council*)

(OPPOSITE BOTTOM). The National Star Centre pool, Ullenwood Manor, Cheltenham. (*National Star Centre*)

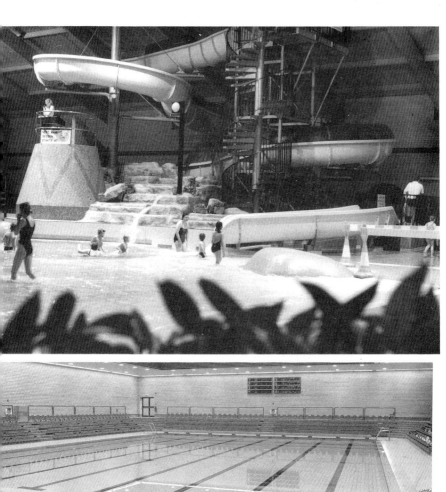

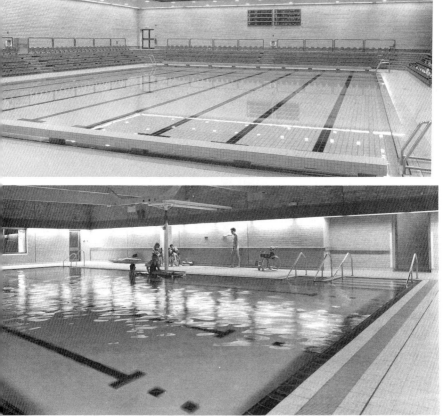

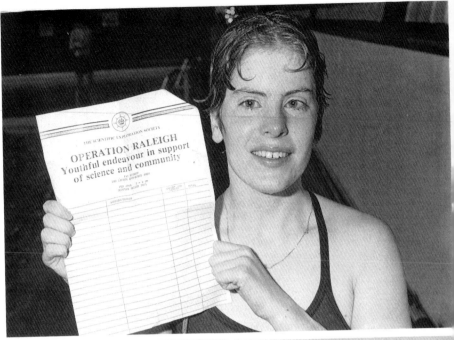

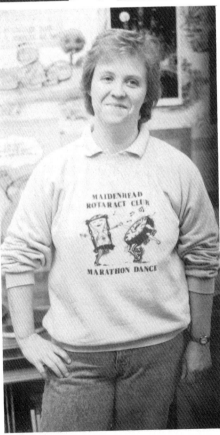

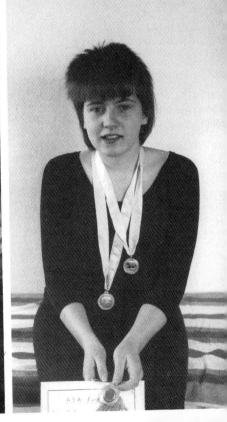

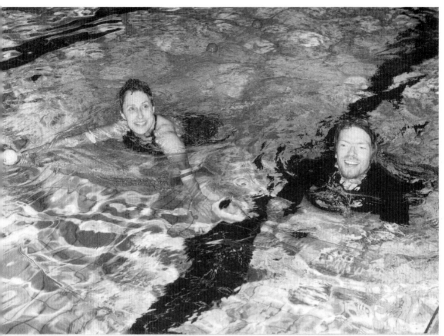

(ABOVE). Jill and Richard anson at the end of her 500-le sponsored swim for Cystic prosis research (Chapter 7). *IC Photos*)

GHT). Jonathan (Chapter 7).

PPOSITE TOP). Fay (Chapter 7) set to go on Operation leigh. (*Harrogate Times*)

PPOSITE BOTTOM LEFT). Anne hapter 7), now a twelve-hour arathon disco dancer.

PPOSITE BOTTOM RIGHT). Sarah hapter 7), with medals and rtificate.

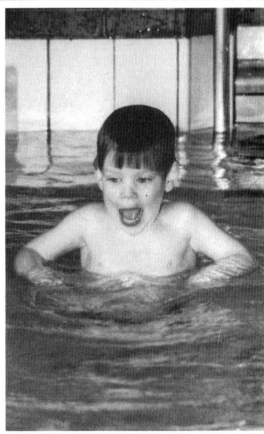

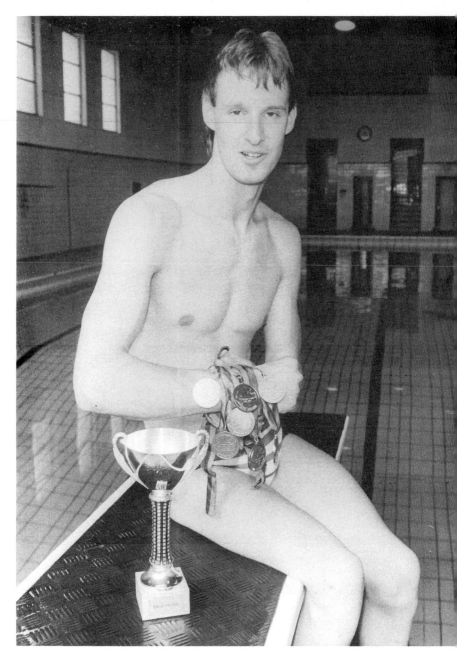

Martin (Chapter 7) one of Britain's leading disabled swimmers, with a handful of gold medals won in international competitions.

vehicle to collect members for a swim and take them home again. But finance should never be the main consideration and must never be a deterrent. The money will come from somewhere!

5. Seek to involve the local newspaper and radio station. Publicity is vital if your club is to get off to a good start.

6. Call an inaugural meeting when all the groundwork has been done. Invite all those you have contacted to date and all the disabled people who you think may be interested. Advertise the meeting but do not advertise for helpers. Helpers of the right sort will materialize; people whom the disabled need, not those who need the disabled. Invite, also, local councillors, the relevant local authority officers, the pool manager and his staff, local doctors and therapists, in particular a physiotherapist with hydrotherapy experience, and representatives from the Sports Council and the swimming organizations for disabled people. Don't worry – they won't all come, but they need to be invited!

7. Make sure you choose an experienced and efficient chairman for the meeting and have a main speaker who knows about swimming and about disability and can convey enthusiasm. The meeting should formally inaugurate the club and elect a steering committee.

8. The steering committee, which if possible should include both able-bodied and dis-

abled members, decides on a club name, badge, rules and structure. On the subject of name, think whether *you* would rather be a member of the Penguins, Otters, Kingfishers, Merlins – or of the Blankville Club for Handicapped Swimmers. The steering committee also sorts out individual responsibilities with both administrative and instructional functions.

9. Decide whether you wish to affiliate your club to one of the national associations, and if so to which. Make sure everyone understands their different approaches before coming to a decision as to which association, if any, will suit your likely membership and your philosophy.

10. The club's swimming instructors must be qualified through one of the recognized national bodies: the Amateur Swimming Association or the Swimming Teachers' Association. The local authority Physical Education Adviser may help with this. Qualified life-savers are essential at swimming sessions. It is preferable that pool helpers should hold the ASA Preliminary Award for Teachers of Swimming for the Disabled and they should also receive instruction in lifting and handling the swimmers safely.

This point-by-point analysis should give some idea of what is involved in starting a swimming club for disabled people. Most clubs develop their own way of organizing themselves, which is only to be expected as some have committees of between twelve and fifteen people with a membership of several hundred, while others are run by two or three enthusiasts with thirty or forty members. All clubs have to take the difficult decision as to what categories of disabled people should be admitted to membership. Safety must be the first priority and without an adequate number of qualified instructors and helpers a club may not be able to accept the responsibility of taking on the full range of disability. Mixing physically handicapped and mentally handicapped people is not fair to either group.

Clubs should also ensure that disabled members have every opportunity to help in the administration, to serve on the committee, and to qualify as instructors or helpers. Evelyn, in her sixties, who suffers from asthma and a blood disorder which causes clotting and resultant trouble in her legs and back, gives testimony to the value of a well-run club:

Five years ago I was medically advised to swim. I could not swim and had a fear of water following being pushed into the deep end as a child. After some weeks of deliberation I decided I had to try, and I joined the Salmon Swimming Club for handicapped people in St Alban's. I was very scared, but in the hands of a very kind, understanding person I soon gained enough confidence to float on my back – this is the answer to fear. I have gone from strength to strength and now do breaststroke, back and front crawl. I still have fear of water, especially if I have not swum for a couple of weeks, but I can overcome it now. I have organized and swum in two sponsored swims for the British Heart Foundation and we are about to do a third. For the past ten months I have been secretary of the Salmon Club, and bless the day I was advised to swim for my well-being. It has given me confidence in many ways – and the best way of summing it all up is that whether able-bodied or handicapped, everyone is the same in water.

A club is likely to succeed if,

a) it understands the needs of its members, ascertained from carefully structured entry forms and tactful questioning, and seeks to meet them.

b) it provides encouragement and skilled instruction, helping its members to achieve the highest standards of swimming of which they are capable.

c) its organizers always have in mind that it is run for the benefit of its members, not for themselves.

d) the happiness and safety of its members are the first priority.

Very important is the club's sense of unity and pride. Track suits, T-shirts and sweat-shirts bearing the club's name and logo are enormously helpful in establishing this. Publicity is also very valuable. Club activities and achievements should be widely known and reported in the local press and radio.

One further point needs careful consideration. This is the time that is reserved at the pool for the exclusive use of the club. Slack times for public use are not necessarily the best times for disabled people and one late evening hour a week may not be the appropriate answer. If possible, the pool should be available twice a week, with one daytime and one early evening session. Each session should be of sufficient duration to allow the more severely disabled ample time to change without being harried or flustered.

Lastly we come to the most important element in the club – the instructors. The teacher of swimming for disabled people needs many qualities apart from teaching skill and understanding of the various disabilities. Among these are sensitivity, adaptability and patience. Constant alertness is essential, especially to ensure that no one is becoming distressed through over-tiredness. Close co-operation with the pool-side helpers is essential; for example, if a swimmer with epilepsy is present, a helper should be nominated to keep constant watch or to swim with him/her, or if a swimmer may require instant medication, one helper should always know where it is kept. The job is demanding but it brings its own rewards. In a recently published article two experienced teachers expressed their satisfaction thus:

> As your club develops you will realize that this is something outside your usual teaching experience. Sometimes you will feel sad, frustrated that you are unable to help more, but there will be a continual challenge to your ability, you will be constantly amazed at the endurability of the human spirit, your pool will hum with happy chatter, ring with laughter and you will give more of yourself than you could imagine. It will be fun!

For some disabled people, however, swimming exclusively with a special club may turn out to be disadvantageous. These are people whose disability is not especially severe or who are perhaps recuperating after surgery and who are also enthusiastic swimmers capable of a good standard of performance. Without the opportunity of swimming with and learning from good swimmers, possibly competing against them, their enthusiasm may become blunted and their full potential never reached. Their situation is improved if the special club operates as a section of an 'able-bodied' swimming club, or is closely affiliated with it. This would allow the disabled to practise and train with able-bodied swimmers and to have the advantage of their coaching. It might also encourage some of the club's regular members to join with the disabled sessions and give instruction where needed. It is sad at times to see competitors at galas for disabled swimmers falling short of their potential through inadequate technique that a lesson or two from an experienced swimmer might easily correct.

In a special club there needs to be assessment from time to time of the needs and abilities of the members. Some, as they improve in fitness and ability, may need to be persuaded to move on into public swimming sessions to make room for new members. In a larger club members may need to be grouped according to swimming ability so that the frailer are not disturbed or intimidated by the younger and more energetic. A club should never become static but must always be ready to reassess the requirements of its members and to adapt to meet them. Some swimmers may deteriorate physically over time; this needs careful monitoring and perhaps recourse to medical advice.

A recent and exciting development in swimming for physically handicapped youngsters has been the formation of the Guillemot Branch of the British Sub-Aqua Club. This was the result of the initiative of Jill Myers who, working with sick children, observed how much at home many of them were in the water. She trained a group of fourteen pupils with various severe disabilities to snorkel and in 1983 took them for a week's snorkelling to the coast of Kenya, repeating this with another group two years later, this time to the Red Sea. The benefits, both physical and mental, were considerable, with youngsters who could barely manage a length in a pool swimming half a mile out to sea with mask and snorkel.

Snorkelling courses for physically disabled young-sters between the ages of eleven and nineteen are now organized in several towns in Yorkshire with the sup-port of the regional Sports Council. The instructors are volunteers from the British Sub-Aqua Club which has formed the Guillemot Branch of which the course participants are members. The club intends to spread the scheme throughout Britain, concentrating on the inner cities where there are a sufficient number of pools and diving clubs.

The object of the scheme is 'to provide a structure whereby under strict supervision physically disabled trainees with medical permission might learn the use of snorkel equipment to experience the underwater world and to enhance their own swimming capabilities.' The emphasis of the scheme is on sport and recreation but it is clear that it also has great therapeutic value. Jill Myers instances the case of eleven-year-old Philip, a spastic child 'with legs as thin as broomsticks' who has never walked and who can stand only with the aid of a frame:

> He was fitted with mask amd snorkel but his mother said it was useless to try fins as he couldn't use his legs. In spite of this we tried and to everyone's amazement he began to thrash his legs up and down in the water using muscles he had never used before. He is now able to snorkel ten lengths of the pool without difficulty. His leg muscles are developing as a consequence and it is hoped he may walk as a result.

Two things are especially noteworthy about this scheme. One is its imaginative quality. Snorkelling is a challenging activity involving not only swimming abil-ity but the choosing and maintaining of equipment on which one's own safety depends. Among the participants on the original trip to Kenya were children with spina bifida, cerebral palsy and rheumatic diseases and a boy who had lost both legs and an arm in a traffic accident. Only the blind, the mentally handicapped and those suffering from fits or seizures are considered unsuitable for this activity.

The other specially notable feature of the scheme is that its inception and success are very largely the work of one person. In this it resembles the Halliwick scheme of the Association of Swimming Therapy – and also the formation of the National Association of Swimming Clubs for the Handicapped. Like James McMillan and Harry Parker, Jill Myers, described by one of her trainees as 'a marvellous woman', has the vision and determination to make a really significant improvement to the quality of life of the disabled children with whom she is in contact.

There have been several unavoidable references to handicap and disability in this chapter. This, if we are not careful, has the unfortunate effect of putting the emphasis on the condition of the person rather than on the person him- or herself. A group of people described as 'asthmatics', 'arthritics', or 'paraplegics' may have little in common apart from that description. People engaged in the same occupation or profession may well share more attitudes and characteristics. Physical handicaps, however, being more immediately obvious, can lead to misapprehensions and mistaken conclusions. It is important to avoid categorizing or stereotyping and to treat each swimmer as a unique individual.

Some disabled people need very special consideration. Many severely handicapped children and young adults spend much if not all of their time in residential schools or colleges, or attend special schools or units daily. Several of these establishments have their own pools and instructors while others may use reserved time at a public pool. For these young people swimming is more than a recreation, sport or fitness-improver; it is an important element in their learning process and helps to instil confidence and self-reliance, as well as giving training in social behaviour. When they leave their school, college or 'sheltered' establishment, however, in accordance with the present policy of integrating severely handicapped people as far as possible into the main stream, they often lose their swimming facilities entirely or find their opportunities for swimming greatly restricted. For these young people joining a special club may be the only solution and if no club is available their needs will not be met.

Endeavour and competition

Most of us, whether able-bodied or disabled, like to have our achievements recognized. Progress in swimming and water skills can be easily measured and several different award schemes are available. Some awards are given for distances covered, either on a single occasion or cumulatively. Others involve the mastery of various skills, including the use of more than one swimming stroke. There are awards for water safety, rescue and life-saving. For certain awards the swimmer himself completes a record card, while others require independent corroboration or the presence of a qualified tester or examiner. Some schemes are open to all swimmers while others are confined to disabled swimmers only.

For many handicapped swimmers, competing for an award that is open to all swimmers provides an extra incentive. The Amateur Swimming Association's Rainbow scheme, a set of fifteen awards for distances from 10 metres upwards swum continuously with no time limit, is easily understood and has something in it for almost everyone. Stronger swimmers may proceed to the Swim Fit and Adult Award schemes for accumulated distances ranging up to 1,000,000 yards within a period of five years, with the swimmer certifying his own returns. The Swimming Teachers' Association has distance awards from 5 metres to 5 kilometres swum under supervision, and also organizes a series of Endeavour Awards for disabled swimmers to be taken in the presence of an examiner. The best award scheme is the one that best suits the needs of the individual swimmer and encourages as high a standard of performance as he is capable of. (Details of some of these awards are given in Appendix B.)

Competitive swimming follows naturally from enjoyment in the water and from the enhanced self-confidence and improved self-image gained from personal performance in the water. Swimming galas are organized by the bodies concerned with swimming for disabled people and can lead to national and international recognition. The organizing bodies have a common aim: to give all competitors, regardless of the extent and nature of their disabilities, a fair chance of success. They seek to achieve this aim, however, in different ways which the aspiring competitor may at first find confusing and contradictory.

There are three main systems of classification for disabled swimmers. In the first of these, swimmers are put into classes depending upon their functional ability. The British Sports Association for the Disabled divides swimmers into five groups ranging from the minimally disabled to the most severely handicapped; a person with no use of his legs but otherwise in a good state, for example, would come into Group 3. The British Paraplegic Sports Society uses eight groups while the British Amputee Sports Association refines further, into nine. Eight groups are also used by the Cerebral Palsy International Sports and Recreational Association and the Spastics Society. Visually handicapped swimmers are divided into three groups for competition with each other, and Les Autres (those with severe disabilities which do not fit into any existing category) have six divisions. For some of these systems Class 1 represents the least handicapped whereas for others it represents the most handicapped, which does not diminish confusion.

The second method of classifying disabled swimmers is by a time band system. This focuses on the ability of the swimmer rather than on the nature of the disability. Swimmers are grouped according to the time they take to swim a given distance. For each distance a number of time bands are laid down (for example: Women 25 metres – Band A up to 22.9 seconds, Band B from 23 seconds to 26.9 seconds, and so on) and swimmers whose times are submitted in advance and who fall within the same limits race against each other. If your time in the race falls outside your time band you are reclassified for future events. This system is used by the British Polio Fellowship and variants of it have been adopted by the Scottish Sports Association for the Disabled and the Scottish Schools Swimming Association. The Special Olympics for mentally retarded adults and children classifies competitors on age and timed performance.

The third method is the one used in galas organized by the National Association of Swimming Clubs for the Handicapped and the Association of Swimming Therapy. This is a time handicap system for which each swimmer submits his best recorded time for a given distance. The swimmer with the slowest time starts at 'Go'; the others start at intervals according to the difference between their times and the slowest. In theory all should finish together if they swim at exactly their submitted time. In practice swimmers are permitted to swim faster than their time by a small margin; if they exceed this margin they are re-positioned.

In time band and time handicap systems swimmers

with different disabilities may compete against each
other and the nature and extent of the disability is
irrelevant. In functional systems events are confined to
swimmers with similar disabilities. One further alternative, preferred by the Mini Olympics for mentally
handicapped people and by the British Swimming
Team for the Deaf, involves neither classifying nor
handicapping and simply puts all swimmers in open
competition with each other. However, it is fair to say
that these competitors may have no physical impairment apart from mental handicap or deafness.

Those who have competed in galas under different
systems say that the functional system gala is more
formal and 'official' with a keen competitive edge. Such
galas are likely to suit the younger and more ambitious
swimmers. In time handicap galas races may take a long
time to complete but they do give an opportunity for the
very frailest swimmers to take part, complete the course
and perhaps win a medal. Whenever possible, the better
disabled swimmers should be encouraged to take part
in mainstream competitions with the relaxation, if
practicable, of any rule that might militate against them.

Details of the various classification systems – there
are at least fourteen of them – are given in a National
Co-ordinating Committee booklet *Classification Systems in Swimming*. As there is much debate and
disagreement about the merits of the different systems,
the concluding section of the booklet, 'A Philosophy of
Classification', is quoted below in full.

> However carefully a system is constructed, there
> will always be some individuals who do not fit in
> neatly to the plan. These competitors should be
> accommodated where possible by agreement of
> other swimmers and officials.
>
> Swimming galas are primarily for the enjoyment
> of the participants and wherever possible the

systems should be moulded around the competitors and not the reverse.

It is always the duty of the swimmers and their coaches to ensure that they have been correctly classified or that accurate times have been submitted. Any query or dispute should be raised prior to the meet, or on the day with the referee before swimming commences. This helps avoid unpleasant disagreements following events.

Competitive swimming can offer disabled people the opportunity to strive for excellence, improve self-image, and enjoy the companionship of their peers.

Behind all the careful organization and planning of classification systems, these opportunities should never be denied the disabled swimmer.

A note on swimming aids

Leaving aside one-to-one teaching methods, buoyancy aids, carefully and appropriately used, can be very helpful. Among the more useful are the poly-otter suit and the bubble jacket which keep the swimmer afloat without interfering with his or her freedom of movement. Those with certain physical conditions may need a particular aid; for instance, some swimmers may benefit from a head support in water. In general, aids which restrict movement should be used as seldom as possible and no learner should be allowed to become dependent on one particular aid. The German 'Swimi' aids have been recommended.

Transit aids, to help the disabled swimmer enter and leave the pool, can be extremely helpful. Especially so is the canvas transit seat used to transfer a swimmer from pool side to wheelchair and vice versa. This helps to preserve the dignity of the individual who does not have to be lifted in an ungainly fashion and also makes

the task easier for the helpers. In pools where the water
level is below the pool surround, mats over the edge
may help swimmers to climb out unaided.

Music may also be regarded as an aid, both to
stimulate activity and to induce a soothing and relaxed
atmosphere. It should never be played so loudly as to
prevent the teacher's or helper's voice from being
heard.

Lucy, a lady in her sixties who is a member of the
Chamwell Evening Club, Gloucester, sums up for all:

> Never did dolphin more delighted play than
>   these;
> Leave in the changing room your aching back and
>   knees.
> The calendar does a backward flip with grace,
> And Youth replaces Age on every face.

5

Exercises in Water

The best general water exercise is swimming, preferably using at least two different strokes. But there are also several simple exercises that can be performed in the ideal environment of water. These may help to increase movement and flexibility in various parts of the body and can be of special value to those who are recovering from an illness or injury. The environment is ideal, provided that it is sufficiently warm, because in water the force of gravity ceases to operate, thus relieving the pressure on painful joints. The density of the water helps to strengthen muscles by providing a non-abrasive resistance to certain movements while aiding other movements where the buoyancy of the water is made use of.

For most of the exercises the body needs to be immersed to within two inches of shoulder-height. This provides firm support and enables you to maintain your balance. Ideally you exercise in water as if the water is not there, and it helps if you have a discreet and appropriate musical accompaniment. A fifteen-minute routine should be enough at first if you are working on your own, building up to thirty minutes if you feel your body needs it. It is very important to pay attention to your body; it knows what it wants and how much it can take. If, for example, it signals pain on a particular

movement then that is a sign to stop. To persist might
do more harm than good.

If you are recovering from an operation or a serious
illness ask advice on an exercise programme from your
doctor or physiotherapist before you begin. Ask for
advice – do not wait until it is offered because it may
never be. Finding out for yourself what is best to do,
and then doing it, is a vital part of the recovery process,
the more valuable because you are taking the responsibility for your own health, not leaving it to someone
else.

What follows is a series of simple exercises in water,
designed to improve muscle tone, increase the flexibility of joints and reduce tensions. No equipment, except
for a float, is needed, but for some movements you have
to make use of the grab bar, or the edge of the elegantly
named 'scum-trough' in pools without a bar. Non-
swimmers may also use a tyre or float in the floating
exercises if they wish. In some pools time is reserved for
exercise sessions, usually with an instructor or under
the auspices of a club. Otherwise choose as quiet a time
as possible. Trying to perform water exercises in a busy
pool leads only to frustration both for you and for
swimmers who have to manoeuvre around you.

1 Marking time

Lift and lower each arm and leg alternately (right
arm/left leg; left arm/right leg). Bring each arm up to
the surface of the water; bring each leg up as high as is
comfortable. When lowering your arms and legs, push
down hard against the resistance of the water.

2 Leg swinging

Hold the bar with one hand and face the length of the
pool. Swing your outer leg forward, back and sideways

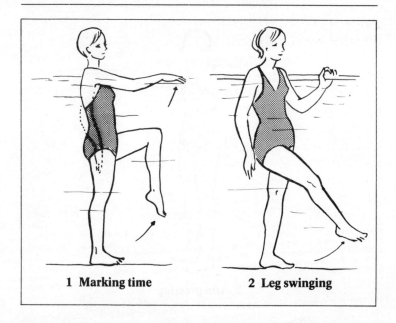

1 Marking time   2 Leg swinging

in sequence. Keep the leg as straight as possible. Then turn to face the opposite direction and repeat the exercise with the other leg.

3 Arm pressing

Face the length of the pool and grip the bar with one hand at arm's length. Raise the other arm to the surface. Pull the arm down strongly to your side. Begin with the thumb uppermost and then change to using a flat hand to increase the effort needed. Turn and repeat the exercise with the other arm.

4 Heel raising

Face the bar and hold it with both hands. Raise your heels so that you are standing as nearly as possible on tiptoe. Lower and repeat several times.

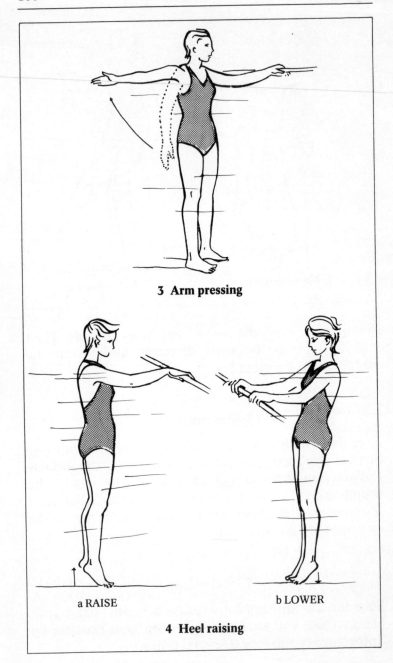

3 Arm pressing

a RAISE

b LOWER

4 Heel raising

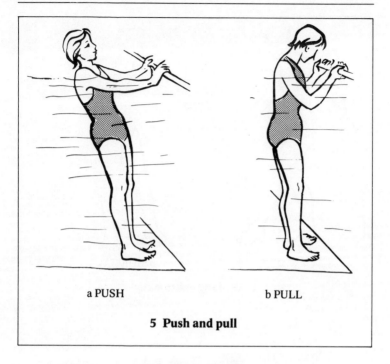

a PUSH   b PULL

5 Push and pull

5 Push and pull

Face the bar and hold it with both hands at arm's
length, gripping either over or under whichever seems
more comfortable. Place your feet close to the bottom
of the wall, with toes touching the wall or within six
inches of it. Pull yourself towards the bar and push
yourself away. This exercise is like doing press-ups
standing up.

6 Walking in the water

Move towards the shallow end of the pool so that the
water is about chest-height. Walk across the width of
the pool: first forwards, then backwards, then sideways
– but don't cross your legs. Walk as normally as
possible, remembering to swing your arms.

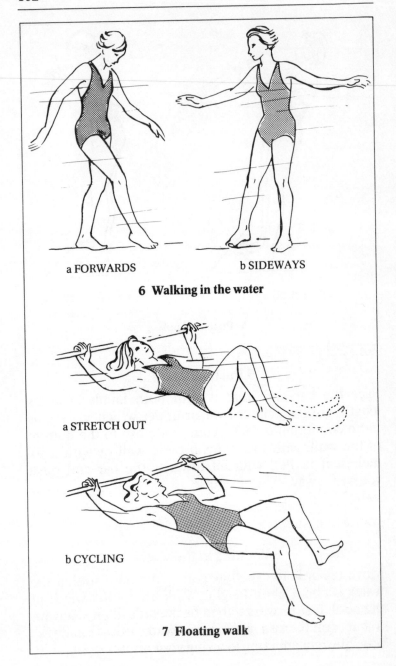

a FORWARDS   b SIDEWAYS

6 Walking in the water

a STRETCH OUT

b CYCLING

7 Floating walk

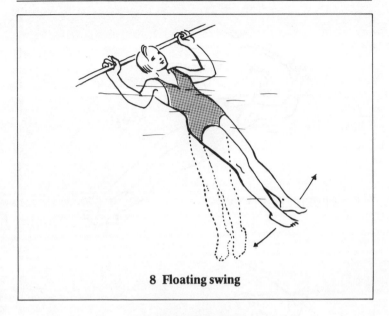

8 Floating swing

7 Floating walk

Hold the bar behind your head and raise your body so that you are floating. Stretch your legs out straight. Now perform a series of walking and cycling movements.

8 Floating swing

Float on your back as in the 'floating walk', holding the bar. Keep your legs together and swing from your waist from side to side.

9 Floating swivel

Float on your back as in the 'floating walk'. Keep your knees together and pull them in towards your chin. Then push your legs down and away from you, still

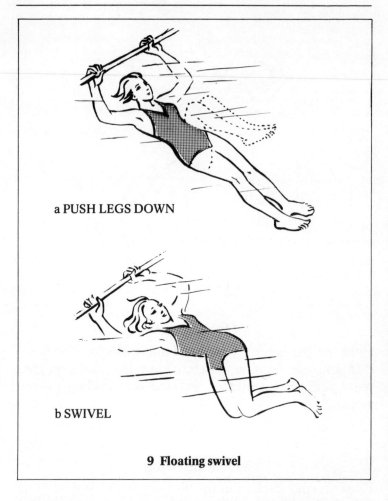

a PUSH LEGS DOWN

b SWIVEL

9 Floating swivel

keeping your knees together. Now, swivelling from the
hips and still keeping your knees together, push to each
side alternately.

10 Floating push/pull

Place a float beneath your head and float on your back
with your feet hooked underneath the bar. Bend and
straighten your knees alternately, pulling towards and

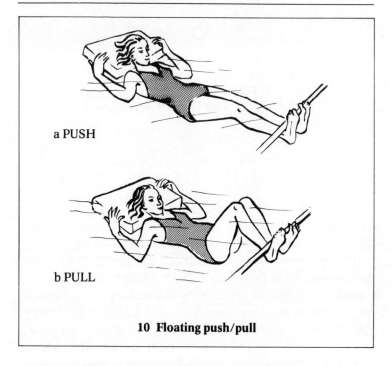

a PUSH

b PULL

10 Floating push/pull

pushing away from the bar. Keep hold of the sides of the float during the exercise.

This is a simple series of basic exercises in water. When you are used to them, try to develop your own variations so that eventually you will have an exercise programme designed by yourself for your own needs.

If and when you find these exercises easy and insufficiently demanding, remember that you can increase the effort by holding a small float in your hand(s) while doing arm exercises or by wearing flippers for leg exercises. Please do not forget, however, that flippers should not be worn during public sessions at the pool.

6

Pools to Swim in

Only recently have the needs of disabled people been recognized in the design and provision of swimming pools. Many of us will remember the pools of pre-war and immediately post-war years: rectangular boxes with a steep gradient, diving boards at the deep end, narrow vertical steps leading into the water which was heavily chlorinated, smelly and chilly. Large windows increased heat loss and noise echoed in the steel rafters. Changing rooms were spartan with minimal facilities and the pre-cleanse area was a wide, unappetising ditch.

For fit, keen and energetic swimmers such pools were adequate, although even they were handicapped by the antics of divers, learners, boisterous teenagers and playful children, all sharing the same water area at the same time in an atmosphere of noisy chaos. Many others, however, were deterred by the experience and although they enjoyed swimming tended to limit their participation to the sea at holiday time or to an occasional dip in a river in the summer. Severely disabled people found it impossible to use these pools at all, being frustrated at many points: access to the buildings themselves, passage from changing rooms to pool side and at the steps from the pool side into the water, which was often too cold for them anyway. These early disappointments put many people off swimming pools for the rest of their lives.

In the 1960s and '70s, however, things began to change. With a general improvement in the standard of living, longer holidays and a shorter working week, more attention began to be paid to the provision of leisure facilities. At the same time a greater awareness of the needs of disabled people began to develop, shown by the passing of the 1970 Chronically Sick and Disabled Persons Act and the 1981 Disabled Persons Act, placing statutory obligations on local authorities to make special provision for them. The Sports Council, the British Sports Association for the Disabled and other organizations with similar interests also made their views and recommendations known. The Disabled Living Foundation came to the forefront of the movement to make sporting and recreational facilities readily and easily available to disabled and handicapped people and published two books, *Sports Centres and Swimming Pools* by Felix Walter, 1971, and *Sports and Recreation Provision for Disabled People*, edited by Neil Thomson, 1984, which gave clear advice and guidance to planners, architects and designers.

As a result of all this, there have been various interesting developments in pool provision and design. Most obviously there is the pool complex: a set of pools under the same roof, each serving a different function. For example there might be a 25-metre competition pool with six or eight lanes and constant depth or only a shallow gradient; a training or learner pool, comparatively shallow; and a diving pit. In 1974 the first 'leisure pool' in England was opened and today there are over forty of these around the country. They are shallow free-form pools with a sloping, beach-type entry, usually with direct access to spectator and refreshment areas. Some have wave-making machines, water chutes or flumes and fountains. The pool side may be adorned with tropical and sub-tropical plants, flourishing in the damp and steamy atmosphere, and coloured spotlights and floodlights are other features. A few of these pools may incorporate a 25-metre straight section but for the most part the emphasis is wholly on recreation. The gently sloping entry makes access comparatively easy for many disabled people who can enjoy sharing the fun with their families in a way not usually possible in a conventional pool.

However, problems still remain, not only in the older pools but also, sadly, in several of the newer ones designed since the recent recommendations for dis-abled swimmers have become known. If financial economy is the prime consideration then some of the design refinements helpful to disabled people may be omitted. Yet in a way this is false economy; generally speaking, improvements for disabled people are improvements for everybody, especially for older people. Swimming is one of the very few sports that can be enjoyed by the over-seventies and if the pools are easy for them to use more of them will swim, thus increasing pool revenues even at concessionary rates.

What, then, are the design features which should be incorporated when old pools are modernized or new ones are built?

Let us begin outside the building. A few parking spaces, a little wider than normal, should be reserved close to the entrance for wheelchair users. Ramps should cover any changes of level between the car park and the entrance, and a sheltered area by the entrance is helpful for disabled swimmers who arrive by coach. Outside surfaces should be firm, not furrowed or covered with loose gravel.

The entrance area should be sufficiently spacious for several wheelchairs, and automatic doors or movable barriers are needed as alternatives to turnstiles. Desks and counters should not be so high that wheelchair-

users cannot reach them or be seen. Corridors throughout should be wide enough for wheelchairs to negotiate
and fitted with continuous handrails. A multi-storey
building requires a sizable lift; otherwise stairs and
steps should be avoided or bypassed by ramps.

Changing rooms need to be large enough for wheelchairs to manoeuvre and ideally should incorporate
both cubicles and open areas with lockers that are
simple to operate. Two or more family changing rooms
with wide benches and their own showers and toilets
are perfect not only for families but for disabled people
accompanied by helpers of the opposite sex. A plinth or
island bench is useful for disabled people who can only
dress or undress lying flat. Large toilets with grab rails
are essential.

Pre-cleanse areas fitted with showers and low-level
jets are greatly preferable to footbaths, but if the latter
are provided a bypass route for wheelchairs is needed.
Non-slip pool-side surfaces with colour contrast tiles at
the pool edge are strongly recommended and texture
contrast is helpful for those with poor sight. The pool
surround should be wide enough for two wheelchairs
to pass each other and a fully equipped first aid room
should open directly on to the pool side. Provision for a
pool-side hoist or lift is needed, preferably one that can
take a person prone as well as seated. While many
disabled people prefer not to use a lift, there are some
who may not be able to enter the water in any other way
unless three helpers are readily available.

The ideal pool hall has as little window glazing as
possible. Large areas of glass increase heat loss and,
more importantly, also create reflections on the surface
which may, as has happened with tragic consequences,
prevent the pool attendants from noticing a bather in
trouble. Natural lighting from above the pool or from
windows set well back from the water area is accept-
able, and artificial lighting should be diffused or

indirect. Good acoustic design keeps the noise level as
low as possible. Suspended ceilings with design features to help backstroke swimmers judge their position
in the pool are preferable to high ceilings that cause
heat loss and echoes.

Lastly, the pool itself. Ideally it should be part of a
complex including at least a main or competition pool,
a learner/training pool and a diving pit. A 25-metre
main pool is the right length for short-course competitive swimming with, if possible, eight lanes. This
enables good-sized areas to be divided off for different
activities. The depth should graduate from 0.9 metres to
1.8 metres or thereabouts. A level deck is preferable:
this has the surface water level at virtually the same
height as the surround and is generally more popular
with disabled swimmers as entering and leaving the
water without using steps is easier. The pool edge
should be marked by contrasting colour and material,
with a handrail or trough a few inches below. At least
one entry into the water should be by a flight of wide,
non-slip, recessed steps with recessed handrails down
to the pool floor. At the shallow end a wide flight of
shallow gradient stairs outside the actual swimming
area, with handrails and a guard rail on the pool side,
makes access easier for handicapped people, the elderly
and young children. The customary narrow ladder-type
steps with skimpy treads and protruding handrails are
dangerous and difficult – sometimes impossible – for
many disabled swimmers. Some training methods for-
bid the use of steps and the swimmers are helped or
lifted in and out of the water. If sensibly designed, safe
steps are installed, however, use of them wherever
possible encourages independence, whether the swimmer is in a club or an open session. These facilities
should be available in the main pool; the learner/
training pool is seldom suitable for disabled swimmers
as there is insufficient depth of water to allow them to

keep their balance.

The water temperature for disabled swimmers should be between 84°F and 89°F. Some pools are run slightly cooler than this and it helps if the temperature can be increased before a handicapped swimmers' club session. Disinfection of the water is a problem and gives rise to many complaints. To keep the water clear, clean and chemically balanced without causing discomfort or distress to the users – each of whom adds to the contamination on entry to the water – is a main preoccupation of pool managers. Until recently chlorine, usually in the form of gas mixed with water, has been the most widely used disinfectant but it is notorious for causing discomfort mainly by irritation to eyes or skin. Owing to its toxicity the Government has recommended that its use be withdrawn. Of the various alternatives, ozone, widely used on the Continent but introduced in Britain only lately, is the most effective, especially when combined with sodium hypochloride, a chlorine compound that provides a residual disinfectant. The system is comparatively costly to install but a little cheaper to operate than chlorine disinfection. The Amateur Swimming Association recommends the ozone/chlorine mix as ideal for heavily used pools, with the extra benefit that it allows the recirculation of air in heat recovery systems and thereby reduces energy costs. There is no smell or taste and asthma sufferers are not affected. Life is also pleasanter for the pool staff who have to breathe this air for hours at a time.

High standards of personal hygiene help to keep pools clean. In this respect, Britain seems to lag behind many other countries, notably Germany and Switzerland. A Sports Council publication has referred to 'the futility of providing pre-cleanse facilities in this country'. In newer pools these facilities have been improved, with fresh-water (not recirculated pool water) showers replacing the old footbaths. All the same, many younger swimmers run through the pre-cleanse showers as quickly as possible, or jump over the footbaths if they can. Apart from being objectionable, low standards of personal hygiene ultimately add to the running costs of the pool and hence to increased charges for admission.

Finally, there is the matter of pool management. Effective management in the interests of all swimmers – able-bodied, handicapped, elderly and the very young – is at least as important as good pool design. Today, time scheduling is common practice at almost all public pools, with blocks of time being set aside each week for adults only, over-forty-fives or over-sixties, length swimmers, ladies only, mothers and babies, disabled swimmers, water exercise sessions and, in term time, local schools. The whole pool may be reserved or sections may be divided off for different activities. Many pools are open from 7 a.m. until late in the evening to accommodate all the demands made on them. Considerate management ensures that disabled swimmers, who have enough to contend with as it is, are not relegated to anti-social hours such as 8.30–9.30 p.m. once a week, but are allocated an afternoon and an evening session a week with ample time to undress and dress as well as to enjoy their swim.

The standard of public behaviour in the pool reflects the quality of the management. Rowdy and thoughtless behaviour is more likely to occur in pools where the manager spends most of the day in his office and the attendants on duty chat to each other in the corners. Positive management ensures that disabled and elderly swimmers are encouraged to use the pool in general sessions and are not always confined to swimming with each other, and encourages competitions and achievement tests for younger swimmers and sets aside time for children's fun and games. In well managed pools dangerous or offensive behaviour is stopped immediately.

There is no doubt that in the last few years there have

been major improvements in our swimming pools and the way in which they are run. Many of them are tributes to the local authority responsible. There are several specific examples of well-designed and effectively managed pools in Appendix A. But indoor pools are expensive to build, maintain and run and there is reason to fear that they may become victims of central government's energetic attempts to restrict local authority expenditure. There is talk of pools being handed over to private enterprise and hence being run for private profit rather than for the benefit of their users. Provided that there are adequate safeguards for the interests of minority users and those with limited incomes this may prove beneficial as it may bring with it a more imaginative approach to the facilities provided and the way they are managed. But the situation needs watching and the organizations representing swimmers have a duty to ensure that swimming as therapy and sport is not sacrificed on the altar of 'fun for all'.

7

Nine Lives

Swimming, like all forms of exercise, cannot be done for you. By deciding to swim for your health you are taking a decision which only you can put into action. You are taking responsibility for yourself, not pushing it off on to a doctor or other therapist. You are taking the first step in a new direction.

Very few are too old or too disabled to swim. At recent galas organized by the National Association of Swimming Clubs for the Handicapped, competitors have included Marie, who propels herself through the water using one frail arm and a flutter of her ankles; Annette, a double amputee who moves through the water like a torpedo; Neil, totally blind; Simon, almost stone deaf; and several swimmers in their sixties and in their seventies. These are competitive swimmers who may have to travel hundreds of miles to take part. Celine, aged twelve, is a typical young competitor who swims at national level. She is paralysed in both legs following meningitis in infancy, and has undergone several major operations. As soon as possible after leaving hospital she is back in the pool, training for the next gala. Swimming will not bring back her ability to walk, but it gives her a physical freedom she cannot enjoy on land as well as enormous enjoyment and a sense of achievement.

If there is a quality that all disabled swimmers share, it is determination. Also notable in competitions and galas is their high standard of sportsmanship. In contrast to what is often seen in professional sportsmen and women, displays of temperament, frustration or disagreement with the verdict very seldom occur. The last to finish may be more vigorously applauded than the first, yet no races are more strongly contested.

The experiences of nine people who have sought new life through swimming demonstrate remarkable qualities of character as well as the success of their search. Two of them are children and in these instances it is their parents, especially their mothers, whose characters are revealed in their particular strength. Their stories are testimony to what can be done if the effort is made.

Martin

The first of these nine people is Martin, aged twenty-six. As a child he was keen on all forms of sport, water sports especially. He took up canoeing at school and alarmed his parents by practising in the bath to see how long he could hold his breath under water. Soon he found that as a canoeist he could compete on equal terms with anyone. Out of his canoe, however, it was different, as Martin was born with cerebral palsy which severely affected his legs from the knees downward and also created problems of co-ordination.

At the age of fifteen Martin began swimming seriously, to overcome his disability and to give him more opportunities to compete. Although he was untaught, his determination to improve and the speed he soon attained attracted attention. Someone at the pool suggested that he should enter for the British Sports Association for the Disabled National Championships at Stoke Mandeville. He went there as an individual entrant, with no coach or team support, and won all his events.

Since then Martin has competed regularly in regional, national and international events organized by the BSAD and the Spastics Society. Coaching helped to improve his stroke technique and in 1984 he swum in the Cerebral Palsy World Games in New York, winning two gold and three silver medals and breaking two world records. In the Sixth International Cerebral Palsy Games in Belgium, 1986, in which nineteen countries were represented, Martin won five gold medals including two more world records and the 'King of the Pool' event establishing him as the World's fastest CP swimmer of the year. He also competes in galas for able-bodied swimmers up to county level.

Martin works as Assistant Head Chef in a large county hospital. He is a qualified swimming teacher (an Associate of the Institute of Swimming Teachers and Coaches) and trains between four and six days a week, swimming about 120 lengths each time. As well as canoeing, he also plays water polo, squash, tennis and badminton, and until recently he was an active member of a sub-aqua club.

Swimming has given Martin freedom and it has also greatly improved his physical condition. By forcing himself to use his legs when swimming he has found that his co-ordination generally has much improved and he is now encouraging other cerebral palsy swimmers to do likewise, even though at first it may limit their speed. His own experience has shown him that disabled swimmers can compete effectively with the able-bodied as well as with each other, but he is critical of some of the ways in which swimming for disabled people has developed. Unless clubs for disabled swimmers are run as sections of able-bodied swimming clubs, promising performers with ambitions to compete are denied the expert coaching and the stimulus of training with high-class swimmers and so may never fulfil their potential. Although these days Martin trains with an able-bodied club he was only invited to do so when he became, as he says, 'someone in the swimming world'.

Martin has now become a powerful driving force in the world of disabled swimming. A main contention of his is that coaching, as opposed to teaching, is grossly under-emphasized and he feels that officialdom generally under-estimates what disabled swimmers are capable of and fails to keep up to date with what is happening elsewhere. As evidence he instances the small number of swimmers in British teams in international competitions, despite their excellent record of success, compared to the numbers from far less populous countries. He is now planning to give up competitive swimming himself in order to qualify as a teacher of disabled swimmers, feeding back into the sport the benefits of his own ideas and experience.

Peter

Although he has never been a competitive swimmer, Peter shares something of Martin's attitude towards the sport. His story, however, is very different.

The time and date when Peter's life changed are etched on his memory: 2.15 p.m. on 6 October 1976. It was pouring with rain when a lorry arrived with a load of steel piping for the firm where he was employed. The piping was fastened in bundles each about fifteen feet long. Peter and his mate unloaded the first bundle and leant it against a wall. They turned away; someone shouted a warning but it was too late; the bundle of pipes slipped and fell, striking Peter down the spine.

For the next two years he was in and out of hospital. He underwent several operations and was eventually left with his left leg shorter than his right. He was also

in continuous pain, necessitating treatment by drugs
which affected his ability to concentrate. The pain and
treatment continue to this day.

Peter was told by his doctor to take up swimming and
the hospital he attended gave him a set of movements to
practise. In the water he found that he was out of pain
and he made the effort to swim regularly, four times a
week.

Peter's wife is also disabled and swims with him.
Their persistence and ability attracted notice, and they
were invited to attend a swimming course at a nearby
town. They agreed, and were surprised to find that the
course was run by the Amateur Swimming Association
for Club Instructors. In the following year they both
went to Southampton University for a pre-teaching
swimming course, which they passed. This was followed by another course, for teaching disabled people.
Next they were asked to teach swimming to the least
able children in a local ESN school. As Peter says,
'Some are deaf, none can speak, all can have fits, so you
have to know how to deal with all of them. We do it for
nothing. People tell us we are mad. We could be.'

Peter and his wife now organize courses themselves.
Each course can take up to three or four months,
including mock and final examinations with all the
accompanying paper work. They also teach normal
children and adults during the week. Peter is now
forty-nine. They have no income apart from sickness
benefit and his industrial pension and they were unable
to afford to attend a further advanced course last year.
Peter says that owing to his disabilities he will never be
able to do a full day's work in his life again. Swimming
keeps him as fit as he can be, preserves him (he says)
from boredom, and gives purpose and motivation to a
life that otherwise might have fallen apart. What he
does not mention is the immeasurable value his efforts
and example are to other people, particularly to those

children for whom otherwise, it seems, life would have very little to offer.

Ann

Ann is a distinguished scholar, a university tutor and lecturer. Although she can walk short distances with crutches and callipers, she is confined for most of the time to a wheelchair – or so one might think.

When Ann was sixteen her spine was fractured in an accident, leaving the lower part of her body paralysed. She enjoyed swimming as a child, although not as the organized and scheduled activity it was at school, and by the age of ten had swum her first mile. The accident, however, put an end to this enjoyment. She was still able to swim in a fashion, and did so while under hospital treatment, but she felt too conscious of her disability to be able to swim in public. For a year she was taken to live by the sea but she never once went near the beach. As she says, 'I was timid about people staring at callipers, withered legs, deformed knee joints; nor did I see how to negotiate sand or pebbles.'

Ten years after the accident, however, she moved to live in Devon and there found that she could actually get on to the beach and into the water on her own. This gave her a pastime that made her feel healthy and was fun. But it was many years before, driven as she says by necessity, she took up regular, serious swimming and brought a new dimension into her life.

Ann was about thirty when she began suffering from painful backache. The physiotherapists told her that her spine was in very poor condition due to long-term damage resulting from the original fracture and from the extra strain put upon it by her efforts to walk, alternating with long periods of immobility in a wheelchair. They held out little hope of improvement but agreed that swimming was the best exercise. For nearly

ten years Ann swam once or twice a week, gradually
building up to forty lengths a time but using only
breaststroke and her self-designed variant of dog
paddle. Then she suffered a setback, damaging her one
relatively good knee. The various consultants she saw
told her to forget about walking and to settle for
enjoying her wheelchair. Ann's response while laid off
work was to increase her swimming to once a day. It
was not easy to get the chair close to the water and
herself in and out of it, but she persisted. 'It was
certainly worth while,' she says. 'Instead of feeling
frustrated and under-exercised, stiff from sitting in one
position all day and miserable because there seemed
nothing much I could do physically, I found that I
could move freely and easily in the water, as well as
being faster than most able-bodied people, which gave
me a feeling of achievement.'

At about this time, Ann met a friend who emphasized
the importance of regular swimming and taught her
how to do the crawl and back crawl properly. Eventually she could swim as well on her back as on her
front, with increased benefit to her muscles. Ann now
swims a mile in about forty-five minutes; the only
problems she finds are shortage of time, the temperature of the water (on occasions) and the thoughtlessness of other swimmers who don't look – or don't
care – where they are going.

Ann enumerates the benefits she has received from
swimming. It has strengthened her back, shoulder and
arm muscles, making both walking and using the
wheelchair easier. It has prevented any recurrence of
backache and strengthened her stomach muscles,
which she uses instead of her legs to propel herself
through the water and to haul herself out of the pool as
she cannot climb up steps. The strength of these
muscles enabled her to walk and use her wheelchair
only a week after a recent major abdominal operation,

to swim after three weeks and be back to normal within a month. Her spine is remarkably supple and strong by any standards, and particularly for someone of her age and with her level of injury. Most of the time, she feels positively fit. Although it is often difficult to find time for swimming during a busy working day, or to drag herself from a warm house in chilly winter weather, Ann is always glad afterwards that she made the effort. 'Aches, pains and tiredness seem to vanish as soon as I get into the water,' she says, 'and mental tension goes too. The swimming hour is even a good time for thinking out those knotty problems that there never seems to be time to sort out during the daily grind.'

Swimming has helped Ann in other ways. It has widened her social life considerably and enabled her to join in other people's activities on an equal footing. This is by no means all. Every year – sometimes twice a year – she travels abroad and swims in the seas, oceans and rivers of the world. She has swum in the Pacific, scrambling somehow up the steeply shelving beaches of Peru, in the Atlantic, in the Red Sea, the Caribbean, in oases by the Dead Sea and in volcanic lakes in Guatemala. Best, she has found, are the gentle, non-tidal waters of the Mediterranean, Adriatic and Aegean – as long, she adds, as you are not obliged to leave everything in a beach hut too far from the water's edge for you to slither on your bottom or walk without callipers. Because of their currents rivers are more difficult; she prefers here to swim downstream followed by a boat, if possible, as walking back to the starting point is impossible if you need sticks and callipers. Ann says that she has overcome her fears about paraplegics being unable to travel or enjoy outdoor activities by keeping her spine supple and muscles toned up all winter by swimming. But basically, she says, 'I swim for fun. The fact that it keeps me healthy too is just a bonus – and, of course, it gives me more energy to enjoy the fun.'

Pam

Pam is twenty-seven years old. At the age of thirteen she was diagnosed as suffering from idiopathic thoracic scoliosis; in simplified terms, curvature of the spine. Since then, until six years ago, her life has been punctuated by major spinal operations. The first of these was in 1975 and it appeared to be wholly successful. For some time she was virtually free of pain until 1978 when trouble recurred.

In the spring of 1979 she saw her consultant, who told her to start swimming – 'to swim as though you really mean it' were his exact words. She did so, gradually building up to a maximum of forty lengths four days a week. This relieved the pain, but it eventually became clear that another operation was needed. This second massive operation took place in 1981. Again swimming was prescribed, this time as a means of rehabilitation. Within a month of re-starting, Pam was again swimming forty lengths a day almost every day of the week.

Unfortunately, the result of the operation did not come up to expectations, and in January 1982 Pam was told that a third one was necessary. This was followed by nine months in plaster with no swimming, not even a bath. Pam noted the date when, the plaster removed, she could swim again – 1 November 1982.

Since that day she has not looked back. Pam swims whenever she can – almost every day. If she misses more than a few days she becomes stiff and the pain begins to return. Swimming relieves the stiffness and the pain, but it has other effects as well. In her own words, 'I feel in myself so much better' after a swim. Often she has had to force herself to get into the pool but afterwards, she says, 'I feel I can lead a normal life and can carry on again.' Swimming has helped her towards solving many problems without conscious effort and coping with the many difficulties that life has confronted her with. One of these is the question of a job; Pam trained as a nurse but was forced to give up because of her health. She tried secretarial work, being a home help, a receptionist – but none gave her the satisfaction she needs. She has now joined the Police Force and is making a success of it.

Pam sets herself the very highest standards. Her swimming achievements are outstanding. Since re-starting in November 1982 she has obtained one Amateur Swimming Association Supreme Award (1,000,000 yards) and is well on the way to a second, swimming front crawl and breaststroke alternately. She has taught herself a whole range of exercises and has taken up running seriously. Seeing her in action now, whether swimming, running or cycling, you would never credit that most of her spine is fused and two metal rods are inserted in her back.

The word 'idiopathic' in the diagnosis of her spinal condition means that the cause is uncertain. What is, however, quite certain is that without her exceptional courage and determination Pam would not have made herself into the fine athlete she is now.

Anne

Anne, aged nineteen, was in training as a nurse at Stoke Mandeville hospital. This hospital specializes in spinal injuries and nursing on the wards involves much lifting of patients. The risk of back injury through lifting incorrectly is well known and nurses are trained to avoid this.

Anne's accident happened off duty when she was putting up posters on the wall of her room in the nurses' home. Unable to get the step-ladder near enough to the wall she stood on the fridge and dressing table. Having finished her decorating she went to put

her foot on the ladder while descending from her perch.
She misjudged the distance, kicked the ladder over, lost
her balance, fell off the fridge and landed heavily across
the fallen ladder, taking the impact on her sacrum. For
a couple of weeks she was in pain and very stiff and she
was forced to take a week off work. No bruising was
visible and the pain subsided. She returned to work and
for a time carried on quite normally until one day after
lifting a patient she felt very severe lower back pain in
the region of the sacrum. Determined to finish her
training she worked on with this pain for a year, lifting
and bending, sometimes not being able to move and
coming off duty in tears, not knowing what to do with
herself.

After she qualified, Anne returned home and decided
that enough was enough. Her GP sent her to a specialist
but he refused even to examine her until she had lost
two stones in weight. Anne had been a keen sports-
woman but by this time she could not even sit comfort-
ably in a chair, and her increase in weight was at least
partly due to her inability to exercise on account of the
pain it caused.

In some desperation, Anne consulted an osteopath,
feeling that at least he could not make matters any
worse. His opinion was that the fall from the fridge had
caused a lot of soft tissue damage which had never been
rested enough to allow it to heal. She was sent to lie on
a firm bed for four weeks. Then he suggested daily
swimming to strengthen the back muscles. Anne began
by swimming for ten minutes a day, gently and slowly,
increasing the time by five minutes each week. She
swam breaststroke, sometimes using only arms or legs,
and backstroke using legs only. To begin with, four
lengths was her maximum; after eight months she could
swim at least forty lengths a day and she went on to
undertake 160 lengths in a sponsored swim for charity.
She began to enjoy most sports again, to hold down a

job and took no painkillers. As she said, 'I wonder if this would be the case if I hadn't started swimming? I dread to think!'

This isn't, however, the end of the story. Ann continues in her own words:

I was soon to find out the hard way – little did I know!

I had psyched myself up so much for the sponsored swim and was so elated on completing it that, somewhere along the way, I forgot the real reason for my daily swimming. During the following six weeks there seemed to be more and more reasons for not swimming; I was too busy, or I couldn't be bothered, or it didn't matter just this once – after all, I wasn't doing another sponsored swim for a while, was I? My back was still hurting but then it always did – and it wasn't really too bad, I kept telling myself.

Then in August I took a beginners' canoe course; two hours a night for a week plus sit-ups to tone up the bulging midriff. My back could cope with the strain, I told myself; if it hurt too much I'd stop. But that wasn't taking into account my pig-headedness . . . and I still wasn't swimming.

The next week was the first of thirteen spent lying on my bed in my room, watching the end of the summer slip away, and losing my job. If anyone mentioned sitting down to me I almost swooned, and fifteen minutes was the longest that I could stand for – if I didn't get acute muscle spasm before then and have to dive quickly back on to my bed. At last I saw a specialist who was prepared to take some action. After two nights in hospital to have a radiculogram (this involves a lumbar puncture through which a dye is injected into the cerebrospinal fluid after which an X-ray is taken) it was found that I had a prolapsed lumbar disc which had been exerting pressure on the ligaments.

Following surgery Anne is now leading an active life again with minimal pain unless as she says, 'I go crazy dancing at a disco'. Three times now she has completed a twelve-hour disco dancing marathon for charity. She has an office job and makes sure that she swims at least four times a week, gradually building up time and distance. She also plays badminton and cycles regularly. 'But I won't again forget why I am swimming,' she says. 'It is too painful a way to prove a point. And the answer to the question "Would this be the case if I hadn't started swimming?" is a resounding "NO!" Moreover I am at the moment President of the Maidenhead Rotaract Club – which I couldn't have been if I were flat on my back!'

Fay

Fay, at the age of nineteen, has just been selected for the final expedition of Operation Raleigh and will shortly be flying to the Bahamas to take part in a series of demanding projects including bridge building, construction and restoration work, scientific research and sub-aqua diving, culminating in sailing back in the sail training ship *The Lord Nelson*. To help towards the cost of the expedition Fay had to raise £1,500; one of her fund-raising exercises was a 100-length sponsored swim in a local pool.

Of the 2,000 young people taking part in Operation Raleigh since its inception in 1984 it was planned that about twenty would be chosen from disabled applicants. Fay is one of these. She is spastic quadraplegic with poor balance and co-ordination, blind in one eye and with limited vision in the other. She was adopted at the age of five when her developmental age was only two and medical opinion was that she would be unable to pass any examinations and would always have communication difficulties. In the last few years Fay has passed six speech and drama examinations with the Royal School of Music, won eighteen medals in the annual Cambridge Festival of Music, Dance, Speech and Drama, has been nominated for the Spastics Society's Achievement Award and has been awarded various prizes for essays and poems. At present she is a student at Harrogate College of Arts and Technology.

Yet possibly Fay's most extraordinary achievements have been in her favourite sports – riding and swimming. Four years running she qualified for the National Dressage Championship of Riding for the Disabled, winning the title in 1984 and being runner-up twice. She was also the youngest rider shortlisted for the national team.

One of Fay's early ambitions was to be able to teach disabled people. She achieved this ambition at the age of fifteen, when she qualified as a Student Swimming Teacher by passing the examinations of the Swimming Teachers' Association, and she now teaches disabled children to swim. For several years Fay has been competing in swimming galas at all levels up to National. In the 1987 National Cerebral Palsy Championships at Stoke Mandeville she qualified to enter in five disciplines of swimming and athletics, and won all of them. At present she is preparing for the sub-aqua element in Operation Raleigh by learning to snorkel with the group of disabled snorkel swimmers already mentioned, the Guillemots. She is also working towards her Duke of Edinburgh Gold award and has recently attended a ten-day drama course for disabled people.

For Fay there is no such thing as disability; it is ability that matters. Her successes are impressive; equally

impressive is her unassuming demeanour and her firm
intent to put back into her sports of swimming and
riding at least as much as she has got out of them. For
many years she was a dedicated member of the St
Christopher Swimming Club at Saffron Walden. When
she moved north recently one of the first things she
became aware of was that there was no provision for
swimming for disabled people in Harrogate. Thanks to
the efforts of Fay and her mother this has now been put
right and this is typical of the positive attitude and
determination she has shown throughout her life.

Sarah

In May 1983 Sarah was nine years old. A bright and
lively girl, she was a good swimmer and had passed a
number of tests. A week before she was due to take her
life-saving certificate she was knocked off her bicycle
by a car and sustained multiple injuries. Unconscious,
she was rushed to hospital. Her level of unconscious-
ness did not change and it was observed that all four
limbs showed increased muscle tone, indicating that
she was suffering from some degree of brain damage.
Quickly she was transferred to the Neurosurgical Unit
at Addenbrooke's Hospital in Cambridge.

At Addenbrooke's Sarah was placed on a ventilation
machine and was fed intravenously. In addition to
severe head and brain injuries she had a severe dis-
placed fracture of the upper shaft of the right femur and
a skin graft operation was necessary to cover a deep
laceration on her right leg. Throughout the time she
was in Addenbrooke's, six weeks, Sarah remained
unconscious.

Sarah's mother, Lesley, is a remarkable woman. She
has two other children, older than Sarah, and she had
remarried less than three months before the accident.
Neither Lesley nor her husband was employed at the

time. Lesley stayed with Sarah while she was in Addenbrooke's, and tells the rest of the story in her own words:

I vowed I would do all that I could to get my child back to normal. I gave myself six months to do this and watched nurses closely as they attended Sarah so that I would know just how to look after her. After six weeks, Sarah was moved to a hospital nearer home. Her level of consciousness seemed to be greatly improved but she was still unable to speak. How was I to know what she wanted or if I was hurting her?

Eventually the cast and traction pin were removed and the physiotherapists commenced trying to mobilize her right hip, which was particularly stiff, and her right knee. Being shown how to do this myself I could help Sarah by making out that it was a game which we were playing. No one had said that swimming or water exercise would help.

I was very anxious to have Sarah home as I was spending a great deal of time with her and knew that once she was home I could think of more ways that would help. The two months in hospital seemed like two years, but at last I was able to take her home. It was just like looking after a small baby again as she was unable to walk or talk.

One thing I did notice was that Sarah loved water and we spent many happy hours in the bathroom – when the water got cold I would just put more hot water in. Then, by chance, I read an article in a magazine about how swimming and exercise in water could help your body regain its strength. I tried to work out ways of getting Sarah to a swimming pool. I myself was, and still am, a little frightened of the water, but I wasn't going to let that stop me.

One day I was pushing Sarah in her wheelchair past the village school, which actually has a swimming pool. Seeing other children in the pool, I took Sarah in to watch. Then a teacher kindly offered to take her into the pool. I watched very anxiously but was amazed to see how well she was doing. It was arranged that whenever I could get her to the pool, someone would be there to look after her. By this time, Sarah was re-learning how to talk and could begin to tell us what she wanted. She could now understand what was said to her but just could not answer back in sentences, but if you mentioned 'water' and 'swim' her little face would break into a broad smile – no words were needed.

It was easy for Sarah to get her balance while in the water. Soon she was able to swim a length of the pool – it was only a few weeks since she had left hospital and I was very proud of her!

One day after coming home from her swim I sat Sarah in her wheelchair to let her watch me prepare the family tea. I was thinking how well she was doing, but I was also worried in case I was rushing her. It was then that I told her – and I don't know why I chose that moment – that some unkind people were pointing at her and laughing at her. She asked why, and I told her it was because she was in a wheelchair but she had not got to let it upset her as they were nasty and cruel. She sat and listened; then to my shock and delight she got up and somehow got out of the wheelchair, called out 'Mum!' and took two unsteady steps towards me. With tears in my eyes I knew then that we would make it back on the long road to recovery.

When Sarah was seen at the hospital a month after being discharged they noted a remarkable change in her well-being. It was obvious that the swimming was helping her greatly. Out of the water Sarah could do very little for herself, but put her into a swimming pool and she was just like anyone else! By this time she was beginning to talk and was walking, though with obvious difficulties because of the shortening of her right leg and the stiffness of the limb.

Arrangements were made for Sarah to have outpatient treatment in a Child Development Centre, and just three months after leaving hospital she attended an Associated School designed for mentally handicapped children. There the physiotherapist would take her into a heated pool. Sarah would tell me it was a big bath and 'it was loverly!' All she looked forward to was her swimming.

Seeing her do so well made me decide to try to overome my fear of water. On our next family holiday all of us went to the swimming pool. One of Sarah's favourite games, we discovered, was to dive in and sit on the bottom of the pool. We, not knowing if anything was wrong, would jump in after her only to find that she had swum away under water.

Since the accident, and despite having to re-learn everything, Sarah has again passed several grades in swimming. A very proud moment was when she represented her school in a swimming gala at King's Lynn. Her school won the Schools Cup and Sarah was awarded a medal. Then just two years after the accident she again represented her school and went to a conference for the disabled at Derby, where she again swam.

Although Sarah can no longer go to discos with her brother and sister, which she found upsetting at first as she loved dancing, put her in a pool and she can hold her own with anyone. She loves

every minute of it and it has done more for her
than anything else I can think of. Once in the water
she is transformed. I am so pleased and proud of
her – she has so much style and grace and to me
she's like a mermaid. Soon, I hope, she'll be ready
to take her life-saving certificate – and this time it
will really happen.

Since the above was written, Sarah has continued to
improve; so much so, in fact, that her Mobility Allow-
ance was withdrawn as she was no longer restricted to
walking less than a hundred yards. She has had to
change schools and as a consequence has lost the
opportunity of swimming competitively, for the time
being at least, and has yet to take her life-saving
certificate. She still swims for pleasure, although, sad to
say, the pleasure is diminished by the behaviour of
other children who draw attention to a minor dis-
figurement, a result of the original road accident. With
regard to this accident in 1983, it is also sad to relate
that the case for liability has not yet come before the
court and the lengthy delay and the uncertainty place
additional burdens on Sarah and her family. Nevertheless she is a cheerful and active girl with a remarkable
talent for writing and drawing, although she has yet to
persuade her mother to overcome her fear of water and
learn to swim.

Jonathan

Jonathan is now five years old. In the first year of his life
he was diagnosed as suffering from cystic fibrosis. This
disease affects approximately one child in every 1,600
born in Britain. It is the cause of two major problems: a
very high susceptibility to bacterial infection of the

lungs and a malfunctioning of the pancreas interfering with digestion and therefore with growth. Untreated it causes irreversible lung damage which in many cases proves fatal. To preserve life, continuous treatment is necessary. Recent years have seen great improvements in early diagnosis and control of the disease; today approximately 75 per cent of children with cystic fibrosis survive into adulthood. As yet, however, it is incurable.

The treatment of cystic fibrosis is threefold: dietary management, antibiotics and physiotherapy. Of these, the most time-consuming and perhaps in practice the most difficult to maintain is the physiotherapy. This has to be carried out daily by the parents, who have to be taught by physiotherapists to assist the drainage of lung secretions.

Jonathan's mother is an excellent swimmer. She first introduced Jonathan to the pool when he was eight months old, but with no success. Following the cystic fibrosis diagnosis she tried again. This time it was different; he took to it at once. Now he can swim several metres, float, somersault both ways and jump in off the low diving board. He swims under water and enjoys himself immensely.

But it is not simply a matter of enjoyment. Having his face in the water forces Jonathan to hold his breath – jumping in from the board leaves him with no choice. This does mean that he vomits quite often; this is no real problem and acts beneficially by loosening mucus and making the subsequent physiotherapy much easier. Swallowing water also helps to loosen mucus by encouraging coughing. Jonathan's mother encourages him to keep his nose and mouth under water as much as possible, tapping him on the shoulder at intervals as a signal to take breath. The frequent changing of body position is also valuable, acting in a similar way to the repeated tipping of the body in physiotherapy.

Jonathan swims twice a week for up to twenty minutes at a time. No claim is made that swimming is essential as a treatment for the disease, but simply that it is proving helpful in its management as far as one child is concerned. Perhaps most important, however, is the contribution it makes to his enjoyment of life. The child with cystic fibrosis does not have an easy time of it and a fun activity which also helps towards his general well-being is of enormous value.

It is interesting to note that the forced expiration technique, where a small breath is inhaled and then forcefully expelled through the mouth, with firm contraction of the abdominal muscles, is strongly recommended by experienced physiotherapists to help shift lung secretions. This way of breathing is employed by many swimmers, especially when swimming at speed. Diaphragmatic breathing is used to relax after one or two forced expirations. Swimmers using a relaxed breaststroke often breathe in this way. It may be that these valuable techniques can be taught simply and effectively in the swimming pool, perhaps as part of a swimming lesson; they can then be readily transferred and employed in the physiotherapy sessions along with the essential postural drainage.

When Jill (see below) began her 500-mile sponsored marathon swim to raise funds for the Cystic Fibrosis Research Trust, Jonathan accompanied her on the first few lengths. He now attends school and continues with his swimming when time permits.

Occasionally he needs a spell in hospital. On a recent visit he had to be put on an intravenous drip and was told that he would have to stay in hospital for two weeks. Jonathan would have none of this. He insisted on being discharged after a few days and went back to school with the drip which he cleared himself when it became blocked with blood.

Jill

With Jill's story we go back to the beginning, to the
opening paragraphs of the introduction. Jill was the
person who was in constant pain, who could not walk
more than half a mile, who wore a surgical collar and
was heavily bandaged, and so on. From the age of
eighteen her life had been punctuated by visits to
general practitioners, out-patient departments, consultants and hospital wards in the endeavour to find a cure
for, or relief from, chronic pain and stiffness. Various
diagnoses were made, queried and replaced by others.
Prescriptions flowed all too freely, the side-effects of
some of the drugs causing further problems and being
responsible for two operations, both of which proved
needless. Advice to keep mobile was constantly contra-
dicted by advice to stay in bed, no easy formula for an
active person who wants to earn her living. As a kind of
compromise there came a new proposal and for many
months she was confined from neck to coccyx in a
plaster jacket. But not long after its removal the pain
returned. A variety of surgical collars was accompanied
by a course of anti-inflammatory drugs which produced
acute stomach pain and internal bleeding. Then
another consultant came up with another diagnosis: a
trapped nerve near the top of the spine. Two weeks in
traction would solve the problem.

The treatment involves the patient lying flat, wearing
a harness around the neck to which a heavy weight is
attached. The idea – a very simple one – is that the
weight will draw the spinal discs apart and free the
nerve. One Friday Jill was fixed into this contraption.
Within a few hours her muscles went into spasm; the
pain was so intense that she was sick. The physiotherapist who set up the device had gone off duty for the
weekend and no one in the hospital was prepared to be
responsible for adjusting or removing it. Jill's struggles

to relieve the discomfort moved the harness out of alignment, which made matters worse. It was a weekend of agony. On Monday morning the harness was removed, but Jill had to stay in hospital for the rest of the fortnight to recover from the effects. Some months later traction was again prescribed, on the grounds that it had not been given a proper trial first time. Despite all warnings the same thing happened, with the exception that there was only one night's delay before Jill was freed. Again it meant several days in bed to recover from Torquemada's treatment.

A new approach was tried. Perhaps the root cause was psychological; a stress condition caused by divorce and re-marriage. Discussions and tranquillizers failed to make any impact, however, and it was back to the rheumatologist and neurologist in turn.

Of the various diagnoses that had been made, one that was often repeated was ankylosing spondylitis, which is inflammation of the vertebrae of the spine, that unless treated early, according to Black's *Medical Dictionary*, 'tends to run an inexorable course leading in the end to complete fixation of the spine'. Whether it was this or whether it was a complex rheumatic condition, early in 1979 the doctors declared they could do no more. Jill was told, in the well-worn phrase, that she would have to learn to live with it and that there would be no difficulty in obtaining a wheelchair when she was ready for one. She hobbled back from the hospital and collapsed in tears.

Two events occurred in the next few months. One came as the result of Jill's visit to her GP to discuss with him the verdict of the consultant. He could not dissent from this, but as she was leaving he called her back and suggested, almost as an afterthought, that she might go to see 'the old fellow who sorts out my back for me'. The 'old fellow' (who has contributed the Preface to this book) soon became Jill's closest counsellor and

guide. He also turned her in the direction of osteopathic treatment, which proved of enormous benefit.

The next part of the story is told in Jill's own words,
from a talk she gave to the British Tinnitus Association
in 1983:

> In August 1979, with my husband, I was seeking
> retreat for a couple of days in the peaceful valley
> of the River Waveney. Even now I can vividly
> recall the unceasing ache of my body from what
> for twenty-nine years has been variously labelled
> as 'disc trouble' or 'rheumatism'. My joints were
> painful to move and all my muscles were
> exhausted and heavy. With my wrists, hands and
> thigh muscles bandaged we arrived to stay for two
> hot, sunny days with Joan and John at their conver-
> ted pub which now houses their small pottery. Into
> the arms of these two dear friends I literally fell –
> crying with fatigue and pain caused by the move-
> ment of the car. But after a good weep and one of
> Joan's soup and cheese lunches, followed by
> home-made meringues, I began to unwind.
>
> The following day was for me, at the age of 47,
> the turning point of my life. As I remember, it
> dawned clear and sunny and while we break-
> fasted we could see the mist rising slowly as the
> sun warmed the fields. I remember the skylarks
> singing with such gusto and joy, and the baby
> rabbits venturing out from an enormous hedge of
> Old Man's Beard to play among the molehills on
> the lawn. I remember so well the contrast of the
> lightness of the day and the dreadful heaviness of
> my body – but the peace is the most vivid recol-
> lection.
>
> After breakfast we set off across the fields. We
> headed for the river which looked so cool and
> refreshing. It was very clear; you could see the

weeds being gently drawn downstream like huge green strands of hair; forget-me-nots grew thickly on the banks and water-lilies bobbed on the surface, with minnows darting between them. Every now and then you could hear a plop as larger fish rose for the midges skimming the surface.

How my body ached in the heat of the day – and how cool and peaceful looked the river!

On impulse then – off with shoes, shirt and jeans and into the water I went. I don't remember when I had last been swimming but I suppose it was on a family holiday earlier in the year. I was no swimmer as such; as a child I had learned with a car tyre tied to a rope and then to a pole held by the games mistress who dragged us up and down the Cam until we could manage on our own. Fired with enthusiasm (I was, after all, Junior Games Captain of my house at the Perse School!) I learned quite quickly to swim the 50 yards or so necessary for house points. From those war-time days I progressed to swimming – or surviving – in the North Sea at West Runton, where 'girls *will* start swimming on Commonwealth Day (May 24) . . .' and so it was, regardless of weather or tide. But after that I swam only on holidays as the local rivers were becoming increasingly polluted.

I cannot find words to describe those few minutes in the Waveney. The day was perfect; and suddenly in those cool, clear waters all the pain left my body. I could move freely; nothing hurt; and for about an hour afterwards whilst my body was drying out I was mobile, light and pain-free. And so it began . . .

Earlier that year the doctors had told me that there was nothing more that could be done. This was a totally negative situation. 'Why me?' I might have asked – but that was pointless. There had to be a positive response – and that quick dip in the Waveney showed me the way. Back home I began swimming daily, gradually building up the lengths. One day an instructor told me about the Amateur Swimming Association Adult Awards for distance swimming. I determined to go for these and at the same time the idea came to me of making use of the time and effort. A few weeks later I began my first long-distance sponsored swim. This was a total of 1,000,000 yards to raise funds for the National Society for Cancer Relief.

Jill finished this swim in a little over a year and raised over £5,000, of which half went in the laying out of a garden at a hospice for cancer patients. She went on to swim 750 miles for the Research and Development Fund of the British School of Osteopathy, followed by 500 miles for the Royal National Institute for the Deaf and the British Tinnitus Association. In the autumn of 1984 she began her fourth marathon, 500 miles for the Arthritis and Rheumatism Council to raise money for arthritis research. It is much to his credit that her rheumatologist of earlier years agreed to launch her on this swim by firing a starting pistol.

It has not all been easy going. One New Year's Eve a mildly inebriated swimmer collided with her in the pool and broke the main weight-bearing metatarsal in her foot. Normally this would have meant putting the foot in plaster for some time. This would have prevented swimming, so the foot was bandaged and left to heal itself, which it eventually did. An accident at home – a sharp bang on the head – caused a brief period of concussion. This was a setback for a time but also a blessing in disguise as the bang acted as instant osteopathic treatment, remedying a long-standing neck problem. More seriously in 1982 there was a malfunction of

her adrenal glands. This caused a long spell off work
and the eventual loss of her job as a university librarian.
It also meant a fortnight in hospital – the longest
non-swimming spell for three years – and then a
determined battle to regain good health.

For fifteen years Jill has been a voluntary hospital
worker with a special interest in rehabilitation. Once
fully recovered herself, she took a training course in
remedial massage, qualified and set up her own practice. Swimming remains part of her programme; if she is
away from the water for long muscles begin to stiffen
and other warning signs appear, indicating that there is
still a risk of some of the old troubles recurring.
Recently she has been swimming competitively, representing the St Christopher Club in regional and
national galas of the National Association of Swimming
Clubs for the Handicapped. Since 1982 there has been
only one interruption of any length in her swimming
when she underwent a hysterectomy. She was back in
the pool on the twelfth day after the operation.

Jill began her fifth marathon, to raise funds for
research into cystic fibrosis, in the spring of 1986. She
was accompanied on the first few lengths by young
Jonathan. This 500-mile stint took just over a year and
gave her a final running total of 3,095 miles of charity
swimming – the distance from Southampton to New
York. As the unchallenged holder of the slowest Atlantic crossing, Jill challenged Richard Branson, holder of
the surface speed record, to join her to finish the swim.
This he did, to make a fitting conclusion to her marathon swimming career.

──The Last Length──

A Conclusion

Much of the evidence of the value of swimming in maintaining and restoring health is what is sometimes rather disparagingly referred to by the medical profession as anecdotal. But there can be no other type of evidence; and in any event anecdotal evidence, if amassed in sufficient quantity, can be perfectly valid in its own right.

This is what the evidence suggests:

1. Swimming is the best all-round exercise there is for restoring, maintaining and promoting health – providing you enjoy it.

2. To be effective, however, swimming must be regular and at least moderately energetic. For greatest effect it needs to be part of a positive attitude towards health, which involves taking major responsibility oneself and includes, for example, sensible diet and avoidance of smoking.

3. Always swim as well as you can, continually seeking to improve your stroke technique,

distance and/or speed. This will provide personal satisfaction and an enhanced self-image.

4. Although facilities for swimming in Britain are improving, in many areas they are still inadequate. More and better-designed pools are needed, and these need to be flexibly and sympathetically managed (see 'A policy for swimming' below).

5. For people with disabilities the evidence suggests that special clubs are very valuable, especially for those in the early or learning stages of swimming. They provide welcome opportunities for those who would be unhappy or need protection in a busy public pool. Wherever practicable and possible, however, integration with able-bodied swimmers should be the aim.

6. The medical and para-medical professions need to be kept fully informed about the special clubs in their locality and should be ready – as in several areas they are – to refer patients to them where it would be helpful.

7. In all matters concerned with swimming for disabled people the interests of the swimmers themselves must be paramount. Organizers and organizations are there to serve the swimmers – as indeed for the most part they do. It must never be the other way round.

A policy for swimming

All public swimming pools should operate according to a considered policy. This will vary in detail according to the facilities, which might range from a three or four pool complex, perhaps incorporating a leisure pool, to a single pool with diving boards. But there are certain general principles which apply to all, in addition to the accepted codes of pool safety and public behaviour.

1. Swimming pools are primarily for swimming. It is not sufficient for an area of water to be provided in which people may do what they choose without reference to the interests of others. In general public times, therefore, part of the main pool should always be reserved for serious swimming.

2. During the week, certain times should be reserved for special interest groups – e.g. senior citizens, mothers and babies, the local disabled swimming club, fun hours for children. These times should not be 'anti-social' but determined after discussion with group organizers or representatives.

3. The highest possible standards of hygiene should be insisted on. This may mean monitoring the use of pre-cleanse areas from time to time.

4. Management should invite local firms to sponsor competitions and fun events occasionally and should ensure that information about swimming awards and opportunities is readily available. This helps to encourage improved performance from swimmers and positive use of the pool.

5. When new pools are being planned, or existing ones modified and brought up to

date, careful attention should be paid to ensure that the needs of disabled swimmers are taken into account and mistakes made in the past are not repeated.

A note on organization

Until recently the Amateur Swimming Association had a National Development Officer for Swimming for the Disabled. This post was funded by the Sports Council. However because of other commitments the Council withdrew this funding, hoping that the ASA would take over financial responsibility for the post. This has not happened and the post now does not exist.

The Development Officer organized courses for teachers of swimming to disabled people and promoted the activity generally. A good officer (and the holders of this post were good) provided leadership, ideas and practical assistance, and many people involved in swimming for the disabled have testified to the value of this contribution. It is regrettable that the funding of this post was withdrawn before alternative funding had been arranged and that the Amateur Swimming Association has to date been unable to make and finance an appointment.

A Policy for Swimming therefore includes the recommendation that a National Development Officer for Swimming for Disabled People be appointed at the earliest opportunity to continue and further develop the valuable work done by previous holders of the post.

Good Pools

Swimming has come a long way since September 1844 when the then Lord Mayor of London called a meeting to form a committee for 'Promoting the Establishment of Baths and Wash-houses for the Labouring Classes'. This committee succeeded in obtaining an Act of Parliament two years later and in 1849 the first municipal baths in London were opened in Green Street, Leicester Square. Within a few years public baths were operating in over twenty towns and cities and several London parishes.

In their way, the larger public bath-houses were forerunners of today's pool complexes with several facilities under the same roof. As well as swimming baths these might include slipper baths, vapour and shower baths, Turkish baths and wash-houses. There might be as many as four swimming baths in the largest establishments: a first-class bath for races and for those likely to travel first-class on the railways; a second-class bath, recommended to be larger than the first but with smaller cubicles and gangways and a shower and 'soap-hole' 'for the use of labourers coming from dirty work'; a third-class bath for boys; and a women's bath. Suggested dimensions for the first-class bath were 100 by 40 feet. The water was heated; one early method was by the injection of jets of live steam directly into the deep end.

Early baths not built under the provisions of the 1846 Act were described as 'more fit for ratting expeditions than for swimming, ill-lighted, badly ventilated, and not often supplied with clean water'. The alternative was open-air pools, favoured by the universities and public schools until the end of the nineteenth century. As the sport became more popular, however, they built their own indoor pools. The conditions therein seem to have been only a little less spartan; Uppingham School's pool was kept heated to a miserly 60°F.

Many of the late Victorian baths survived until well into the present century. The pools which supplemented or replaced them were on a smaller scale; the class distinctions and the separate pools for women disappeared, and small learner or children's pools were introduced. In general diving boards remained as an adjunct to the deep end, which was made far deeper than would otherwise be necessary. It was some time before it was realized that heating the air was as important as heating the water and that slippery white tiles were not the only materials suitable for the pool and its surround.

The fifties and sixties saw many changes in approach to pool design, not all of them very practical. There was a greater use of glass in pool halls, resulting in excessive heat loss and troublesome, sometimes dangerous, reflections on the water surface. Amenities generally were improved although there was no realization that disabled people might want or need to use the pool.

However, in the last twenty years there have been significant changes in the thinking relative to pool provision and Britain is now beginning to catch up with countries such as Germany and Switzerland where this provision has been both more lavish and more imaginative in recent times.

Today there are about 2,500 public swimming pools operated by local authorities in the United Kingdom and Eire, of which only 157 are outdoor pools. In addition there are some 6,000 school pools, 300 pools belong to independent schools, universities and colleges, and about 1,000 pools owned by hotels and various organizations. There are also over forty free-form leisure pools in the larger towns and cities and popular holiday resorts. Recent developments include the introduction of slides and flumes (water slides), the provision of saunas, sun-ray treatment beds, 'fitness suites' and similar amenities, and the installation of movable floors and booms to divide off sections of the pool.

A good example of modern pool design is the Crown Pools complex, Ipswich, opened in 1984. This comprises a 25-metre, eight-lane competition pool, a free-form leisure pool with sloping beach areas, wave machine, waterfall and fountain, and a small teaching pool. There is seating for 600 spectators around the competition pool and this area can be divided off by soundproof curtains. Tropical and sub-tropical plant beds surround the leisure and training pools which are illuminated by an impressive array of spotlights and floodlights. To increase income, this area can be rented out for fashion shows and similar events. Disabled swimmers have their own changing rooms and easy wheelchair access to the pool side. The complex combines facilities for competitive, serious and recreational swimming under one roof. Diving facilities are available in an older pool close by; this pool may also be hired by swimming clubs and is used regularly by the local club for handicapped swimmers. The management promotes full use of the pools with plenty of competitive events and achievement tests for younger swimmers, some of them sponsored by local firms, and ensures that splashers and fun-lovers do not conflict with serious swimmers. The complex is centrally situated with ample car-parking adjacent.

Other notable examples of pool design include the Guildford Sports Centre, 1972, the Barnet Copthall complex, Hendon, 1977, with three pools much used for top-class competitive swimming and diving, and the North Devon Leisure Centre pool in Barnstaple. The Dolphin Leisure Centre in Darlington, 1982, has four pools under the one roof and also houses a remarkable range of other activities in a building designed with exceptional ingenuity. The Bath Leisure Centre incorporates a pool designed with disabled swimmers in mind, lined with tiles imported from Germany which expand and contract with temperature changes. The heat can be increased by 8–10°F overnight should it be necessary.

All the requirements for severely disabled swimmers may be seen in the pool at the National Star Centre for Disabled Youth, near Cheltenham. This is 16.6 by 9 metres, sloping from 0.9 to 1.45 metres in depth. It is a deck level pool with non-slip, tiled surround in contrasting textures and colours. There are four means of entry into the water: a flight of wide, shallow steps and a flight of rather steeper steps, both with handrails, leading in from outside the swimming area; a set of conventional vertical steps recessed into the surround; and an efficient, easily operable hoist that enables entry either prone or seated. Submersible wheelchairs are available and these can be lowered into the pool down the shallower steps. The hall has a low ceiling and lighting which creates no reflections. Bounced ceiling lights can create changes of mood for recreational swimming and underwater lighting illuminates the pool floor. There is a warm and pleasant atmosphere in the pool hall, helping to eliminate distractions (often caused by jazzy colour schemes) and to foster confidence in the environment. Almost all the features here would be of value in the design of a public pool.

An interesting recent development is the Kingfisher

Leisure Pool at Sudbury. Since 1939 this Suffolk town of about 12,000 inhabitants had been served by an open air pool only. To replace it the District Council decided to build a leisure pool on a central site. This was opened in the summer of 1987. The council, which had hitherto employed only one pool staff member, handed over the management and operation of the pool to a private company for a fixed fee, the council retaining responsibility for loan charges and external and structural maintenance.

The single large pool, designed by the Charter Partnership, incorporates a 25-metre, six-lane competition area and a gently shelving leisure pool with waterslide, fountains, waterfall and small toddlers' pool. A spiral flume leads into a separate splashdown pool. There is a large 'unisex' changing area with cubicles, lockers and big cubicles for family or disabled people's use. Among other features are a health suite, conditioning room, solarium and good refreshment facilities. Especially impressive is the spacious foyer with its emphasis on ease of entry rather than, as many pool foyers, on making entry as tight and difficult as possible.

Much thought has been given to the use of the pool by disabled people and improvements are continually being made. One grateful user wrote, 'I found to my surprise that the doors were wide enough for a wheelchair, there were toilets for the disabled and three special changing rooms for disabled people's use, big enough for a wheelchair and still room to swing legs around, and an elevator to the top floor plus many other features.' Submersible wheelchairs can be taken into the pool until the depth is sufficient for the occupant to swim.

One feature of the Sudbury pool, however, highlights the problems of compromise. A wave machine is installed, which operates at certain scheduled times and is a great attraction. This unfortunately necessitates that the level of the water in the six-lane swimming area is far below the level of the surround, making it very difficult for anyone to get out without using the steps, and impossible for most disabled people. This could present great difficulty in an emergency where it was impractical to leave the water through the leisure area. However, with energetic and imaginative management, closed-circuit television, keen supervision and full control of all the pool's facilities from a constantly manned central console, emergencies here, should any occur, are likely to be handled promptly and effectively.

Sudbury's combination of public and private enterprise, also in operation at a handful of other centres, may turn out to be the route to follow for the provision of the best facilities for all at charges that are not prohibitive.

Appendix B

Some Swimming Awards

These awards are available to everyone over the age of eighteen – able-bodied and handicapped alike. Badges and certificates are awarded for nominal charges.

Amateur Swimming Association Adult Award Scheme

For these awards you obtain a card from the ASA representative (see Useful Addresses at the end of this book) and complete it yourself after each swim. You record the date when you commenced the scheme, the date of each swim, the distance of the swim, and the running total. The running totals entitle you to awards as follows:

1. Bronze Award: 20,000 yards (18,290 metres)   in six months
2. Silver Award: 35,000 yards (32,000 metres)   in twelve months
3. Gold Award: 65,000 yards (59,440 metres)   in two years
4. Diamond Award: 150,000 yards (137,160 metres)   in three years
5. Supreme Award: 1,000,000 yards (914,440 metres)   in under five years

You may obtain a lapel badge and a costume badge for each stage you complete.

For these awards you don't have to swim non-stop at each session; what counts is the total number of lengths completed in each swim. Nor do you need an examiner or witness; if you don't record accurately, the only person you are cheating is yourself! In a way, this type of distance swimming is the equivalent of jogging – except that it provides a fuller exercise for the whole body. The awards provide a valuable incentive and the distances are well within the capacity of the great majority of swimmers.

There are problems with length swimming if the only times you can get to the pool are when it is crowded. But if a few of you can get together at the same time you should ask the pool manager if he would close off a couple of lanes for length swimmers. Managers usually will do whatever they can to help.

Swim Fit Awards

These operate similarly to the Adult Awards but with no time limits. Running totals are kept in miles, yards or metres, and style or speed do not come into account. Swimmers keep their own record cards. Badges are awarded for the following distances:

10 miles	(17,600 yards or 16,095 metres)
20 miles	(35,200 yards or 32,190 metres)
40 miles	(70,400 yards or 64,380 metres)
80 miles	(140,800 yards or 128,760 metres)
100 miles	(176,000 yards or 160,950 metres)
150 miles	(264,000 yards or 241,425 metres)
200 miles	(352,000 yards or 321,900 metres)
250 miles	(440,000 yards or 402,375 metres)
300 miles	(528,000 yards or 482,850 metres)
350 miles	(616,000 yards or 563,325 metres)
400 miles	(704,000 yards or 643,800 metres)
450 miles	(792,000 yards or 724,275 metres)
500 miles	(880,000 yards or 804,750 metres)

There is no age limit to these awards.

Amateur Swimming Association Rainbow Award Scheme

This scheme is organized together with the English Schools' Swimming Association. It is available for swimmers of all ages. Costume badges of different colours are awarded for distances swum continuously without any time limit. The distances are carefully graduated as follows:

10 metres – Purple	1,500 metres – Gunmetal
25 metres – Red	2,000 metres – Orange
50 metres – Blue	3,000 metres – Bordeaux
100 metres – Green	4,000 metres – Citron
200 metres – Yellow	5,000 metres – Cypress
400 metres – Ceramic blue	7,500 metres – Olive green
800 metres – Nut brown	10,000 metres – Grotto blue
1,000 metres – Meyron rose	

The swim should be witnessed by an ASA affiliated club official, swimming teacher or coach, school teacher or similar – in practice, a permanent member of the pool staff will normally qualify.

The same two organizations also offer Water Skills awards. These come in six grades, with ten tests in each, and are open to all swimmers. Again, a wide range of examiners may assess for these awards.

More demanding are the ASA Swimming Challenge Awards – bronze, silver and gold. These involve using more than one stroke (for the Gold Award three strokes are required) with uninterrupted swimming up to 800 metres and the performance of a range of manoeuvres. These awards would not be suitable for many handicapped swimmers.

The Swimming Teachers' Association Awards

The STA awards Adult Swimming Achievement Certificates. To qualify you have to pass graded tests in the presence of an STA examiner, and a small fee is payable.

The tests are as follows:

Grade 1: Bronze Award

1. Enter the water unaided without using steps.
2. Demonstrate the ability to regain a standing position from swimming (a) on the back (b) on the front.
3. While standing in chest-deep water, retrieve an object from the bottom of the pool unaided.
4. Push off into deep water and swim along the pool side using any front stroke for a distance of 5 metres.
5. Push and glide, holding the glide position for ten seconds.
6. Climb unaided from the water without using the steps. (This may be performed at the shallow or deep end of the pool.)
7. Swim a distance of 5 metres using any backstroke then, without touching the bottom or sides of the pool, roll into a front swimming position and continue in the same direction for a further 5 metres.
8. Perform back paddle (sculling with the hands, flutter kick with the feet) in deep water for 10 metres.
9. Tread water for thirty seconds.
10. Swim 25 metres, any backstroke other than back paddle.

Grade 2: Silver Award

1. Enter the water by a jump or dive unaided.
2. Climb out of deep water without using the steps.

3. From the pool side, help someone safely from deep water.
4. Swim to retrieve an object from the bottom of the pool in a water depth of at least 1 metre.
5. Tread water for one minute.
6. Perform a head first entry into deep water and glide to surface.
7. Perform a motionless back float, and show how the repositioning of the arms affects the body position in the water.
8. Demonstrate the ability to propel oneself for 5 metres, in the supine position using arms only (a) head first (b) feet first.
9. Swim a distance of 100 metres using three different strokes (one of which must be a backstroke) from the following: each stroke must be swum continuously for at least 25 metres. (Breaststroke, sidestroke, front crawl, back crawl, English backstroke.)
10. Demonstrate the ability to perform expired air resuscitation.

Grade 3: Gold Award

1. Jump or plunge into the water from a height of 1 metre.
2. Swim 50 metres.
3. Climb unaided from deep water without using the steps (these three tests must be performed clothed; male: shirt and shorts, or long pyjamas; female: skirt and blouse, or long pyjamas).
4. Perform a plunge dive or plain header from the pool surround. Legs must be straight at the knees, and feet together on entry.
5. Perform a pendulum float from supine to

prone position, showing how the arms and
head are used to regulate the body position
in the water.

6. Swim to retrieve an object from the bottom
of the pool in a water depth of at least 1.5
metres.

7. Tread water for three minutes.

8. In an efficient manner, assist a conscious
but passive subject from the centre of the
pool on to the pool surround.

9. Give a practical demonstration of expired
air resuscitation, then place the subject in
the coma position.

10. Swim 400 metres using three different
strokes, one of which must be a backstroke.
Each stroke must be performed
continuously for at least 100 metres. Strokes
to be selected from the following:
Breaststroke, sidestroke, front crawl, back
crawl, English backstroke.

Having obtained your STA Gold Award you are
eligible to enter for a series of advanced tests leading to
the Performer's Diploma.

The STA also has a series of awards available to
disabled swimmers. This is the Endeavour Series; there
are four stages, as follows:

The Basic Endeavour Award

This is for swimmers of all ages and abilities who have
proved that by endeavour they have succeeded in
reaching any given standard. Hence a handicapped
child who has managed a few strokes 'as a direct result
of constant practice combined with tenacity of purpose'
would qualify, at the discretion of an authorized STA
examiner.

Bronze Endeavour
1. Breathing control. Submerge the face and exhale under the water once only.
2. Flotation. Demonstrate the ability to float for a minimum period of fifteen seconds.
3. Propulsion. Travel a measured distance of 10 metres by the use of any stroke.
4. Watermanship. Demonstrate any one of the following three exercises:
   a) Recover an object from the water of at least waist-depth.
   b) Change body position, without assistance, from a prone position to supine, or supine position to prone.
   c) Propel a floating object for a distance of 2 metres.

Silver Endeavour
1. Breathing control. Submerge the face and exhale under water, repeating four times.
2. Flotation. Demonstrate the ability to float in a relaxed manner for a minimum of twenty seconds.
3. Propulsion. In any competent manner, swim a distance of 25 metres.
4. Watermanship. Demonstrate any two of the following four exercises:
   a) Enter the water unaided and recover to a swimming position.
   b) From a swimming position, in waist-deep water, recover an object from the bottom of the pool.
   c) Swim a distance of 25 metres to a floating object and return with the object to the starting-point.
   d) With the body in a sitting or back lying position, rotate on the surface of the

water (as a record turntable) for two complete revolutions by the use of hands and/or feet, as desired.

Gold Endeavour

1. Breathing control. Submerge the face and exhale under water. Repeat seven times.
2. Flotation. Either (a) or (b).
   a) Float for a minimum of thirty seconds without limb movements.
   b) Maintain a vertical position in the water for sixty seconds.
3. Propulsion. Either (a) or (b).
   a) Swim 100 metres in the prone and 25 metres in the supine positions.
   b) Swim 100 metres in the supine and 25 metres in the prone positions.
4. Watermanship. Choose any three of the following five exercises:
   a) Enter the water unaided and recover to a swimming position. Swim a distance of 10 metres, then leave the water unaided.
   b) From a swimming position in chest-deep water, recover an object from the bottom of the pool.
   c) Tow an able-bodied subject a distance of 10 metres.
   d) Whilst swimming a distance of 25 metres demonstrate the ability to change position from prone to supine and back again.
   e) Whilst swimming a distance of 25 metres, demonstrate the ability to change position from supine to prone and back again.

All the STA awards are part of the organization's International Swimming Teaching Awards Programme and annotated leaflets are readily available from association members and at swimming pools. There are also awards for Distance Swimming, Watermanship, Survival and Synchronized swimming.

The Scottish Amateur Swimming Association Awards

The Beaver Awards of the Scottish Amateur Swimming Association are valuable for young swimmers with special needs. They are intended for pupils of recognized Special Schools or for those whose handicap means that they cannot swim on equal terms with able-bodied swimmers. Twenty-eight skills are tested with a point being awarded for each. There are four grades of award so that a swimmer who can perform any five skills obtains Grade 1 and may proceed, until by mastering twenty skills he arrives at Grade 4.

Full details of the Beaver Awards are obtainable from the Secretary of the National Award Scheme, 44 Frederick Street, Edinburgh.

Useful Addresses

Swimming Organizations

Amateur Swimming Association
(ASA)
Harold Fern House,
Derby Square,
Loughborough,
Leicestershire LE11 0AL

Institute of Swimming Teachers
and Coaches (ISTC)
Lantern House,
38 Leicester Road,
Loughborough,
Leicestershire LE11 2AG

Swimming Teachers
Association (STA)
Anchor House,
Birch Street,
Walsall WS2 8HZ

Association of Swimming
Therapy (AST)
Secretary,
Treetops,
Swan Hill,
Ellesmere,
Salop SY12 0LZ

National Association of
Swimming Clubs for the

Handicapped (NASCH)
Administrator,
84 Botley Road,
Park Gate,
Southampton SO3 7BA

British Sports Association for
the Disabled (BSAD)
Hayward House,
Barnard Crescent,
Aylesbury,
Bucks HP21 8PP

Scottish Sports Association for
the Disabled
(Mr R. Brickley, Fife Institute of
Physical & Recreational
Education)
Viewfield Road,
Glenrothes,
Fife KY6 2RA

Welsh Sports Association for
the Disabled
c/o Sports Council for Wales,
Sophia Gardens,
Cardiff CF1 9SW

The Sports Council
16 Upper Woburn Place,
London WC1H 0QP

Sports Council for Northern
Ireland
2a Upper Malone Road,
Belfast BT9 5LA

Scottish Sports Council
1 St Colme Street,
Edinburgh EH3 6AA

Sports Organizations for Specific Disabilities

British Amputee Sports
Association (BASA)
Dr G. Thomas,
c/o Hayward House,
Barnard Crescent,
Aylesbury,
Bucks HP21 8PP

British Deaf Sports Council
Swimming Section:
Mr E. Webb,
9 Windsor Grove,
Ashton-under-Lyne,
Lancs

British Paraplegic Sports
Society
Sir Ludwig Guttmann Sports
Centre,
Stoke Mandeville,
Harvey Road,
Aylesbury,
Bucks HP21 8PP

British Les Autres Association
239a Thomas Close,
Southgate,
Runcorn,
Cheshire

British Polio Fellowship
Bell Close,
West End Road,
Ruislip,
Middlesex HA4 6LP

Royal National Institute for the
Blind
(British Association for
Sporting & Recreational
Activities for the Blind)
224 Great Portland Street,
London W1N 6AA

The Spastics Society (Sport &
Recreation Section)
Fitzroy Square,
London W1P 5HQ

Special Olympics UK
Michael House,
47 Baker Street,
London W1

The Asthma Society
12 Pembridge Square,
London W2 4EH

United Kingdom Sports
Association for People with
Mental Handicap
c/o The Sports Council,
16 Upper Woburn Place,
London WC1H 0QP

Mini Olympics
23 Mansfields,
Writtle,
Chelmsford,
Essex

Useful Books

These books should be available from bookshops and/or public libraries. Those published by the Amateur Swimming Association may be obtained from the association at Harold Fern House, Derby Square, Loughborough, Leics. LE11 0AL.

Adapted Aquatics, American National Red Cross (Doubleday & Co., New York 1977). A comprehensive manual on swimming for disabled people.

The ASA Guide to Better Swimming, edited by Rick Cross (Pan Books 1987). A compendium of advice by a team of experienced coaches.

Competitive Swimming Manual for Coaches and Swimmers, James E. Counsilman (Pelham Books, London 1978).

The Handbook of Swimming, David Wilkie & Kelvin Juba (Pelham Books, London 1986). Clearly written and very well-illustrated, with much interesting information about the sport.

The Science of Swimming, James E. Counsilman (Pelham Books, ninth impression 1982). The swimmers' bible.

The Science of Teaching Swimming, Mervyn L. Palmer (Pelham Books, London, reprinted 1984). Primarily for swimming teachers, this is a well-researched study. Illustrated with drawings.

Splash, David Wilkie & Kelvin Juba (Stanley Paul, London 1982). A sound introductory book based on a TV programme.

Sports & Recreation Provision for Disabled People, edited by Neil Thomson, Disabled Living Foundation, 1984 (DLF Sales, Book House, 45 East Hill, Wandsworth, London SW18 2QZ). A thorough and authoritative survey.

Sports Centres and Swimming Pools, Felix Walter, Disabled Living Foundation, 1971 (as above). Replaced by title above but remains a valuable survey.

Swim for Fitness, Marianne Brems (Chronicle Books, San Francisco, reprinted 1985). A useful practical manual illustrated with drawings.

Swimming, John Verrier (Crowood Press, Marlborough 1985). A straightforward instructional book especially suitable for younger swimmers.

Swimming Medicine vol 4. Proceedings of the Fourth International Congress, Stockholm 1978. For knowledgeable specialists.

Swimming for the Disabled, Association of Swimming Therapy (EP Publishing, Wakefield 1981). A full account of the Halliwick method and the working of the Association.

Swimming for Schools, A. H. Owen (Pelham Books, London fifth impression 1979). A comprehensive manual for swimming teachers.

The Teaching of Swimming, Amateur Swimming Association (twelfth edition 1985). Frequently revised and updated. An authoritative handbook.

Teaching of Swimming for those with Special Needs, Amateur Swimming Association. A set of papers from Sunderland Polytechnic covering most aspects of the subject. First published 1984 but to be revised and illustrated in the light of comments.

Yoga and Health, S. Yesudian and E. Haich (Unwin paperbacks, London, reprinted 1984).

The National Co-Ordinating Committee on Swimming for the Disabled publish six booklets: *Forming a Club, Lifting and Handling, Swimming and Epilepsy, Facilities, Medical Considerations*, and *Classification Systems in Swimming*. They can be obtained from the Sports Council.

The Register of Swimming Clubs and Organized Swimming Sessions for Handicapped People can be obtained from the NASCH Administrator, 84 Botley Road, Park Gate, Southampton SO3 7BA.

The following periodicals often include useful articles and information on aspects of swimming, including swimming for disabled people:

The Swimming Times, Amateur Swimming Association, monthly

The Swimming Teacher, Swimming Teachers' Association, monthly

In the Swim, Institute of Swimming Teachers and Coaches, quarterly

—Acknowledgements—

Many people have helped in the writing of this book; indeed without the swimmers who completed questionnaires there would be no book at all. I have a special debt of gratitude to those who told their personal stories in full and who readily agreed to share their experiences with others. I am also grateful to the eighty practising osteopaths, all members of the Register of Osteopaths of the British School of Osteopathy, who supplied answers to my questions.

Others who helped in various ways, often giving up much of their time in interviews and correspondence, include Ken Black of the National Star Centre for Disabled Youth, Paul Barber, sometime National Development Officer of the Amateur Swimming Association, Mrs Edna Jones, Martin Mansell, Mrs Muriel Kenworthy, Dr Joan Martin, Mr C. J. Becket of Pinderfields Hospital, Mr John Blanchard, the Principal of SENSE's residential home at Market Deeping, Mr Nigel Palastanga of the Physiotherapy School, Addenbrooke's Hospital, Mrs Phyl McMillan, and officers of the Amateur Swimming Association, the Swimming Teachers' Association, the National Association of Swimming Clubs for the Handicapped, the Association of Swimming Therapy and the Disabled Living Foundation. The managers and assistant managers of many swimming pools gave invaluable help and I would make special mention of those at Darlington Dolphin Centre, Ipswich Crown Pools, Barnet Copthall, Bath Leisure Centre, Sudbury Kingfisher Pool and North Devon Leisure Centre. I would emphasize that all opinions expressed, unless directly quoted, are my own.

Quotations from *The Science of Swimming* by James E. Counsilman are printed by kind permission of Pelham Books Ltd, and from *Doran; Child of Courage* by kind permission of Linda Scotson and William Collins Sons & Co Ltd. The Health Education Council generously allowed the reproduction of the 'S-Factor Score' table from the booklet *Looking after Yourself*. Details of the various awards are given by permission of the various swimming organizations.

Since I began researching for *Swimming for Life*, Jill has swum the equivalent distance from Southampton to New York, 3,095 miles, for charity. Her contribution – not simply to the book but far more importantly to the health and happiness of many others whom she has encouraged to swim regularly or who have followed her example – has been incalculable.

Index